Live Well...Be Healthy

Live Well...Be Healthy

Dr John Marsden
& Alison Dillon

This book is published to accompany the third television
series of *Body Hits*, made by the BBC's Popular
Features Unit for BBC3. The first series was broadcast
on BBC3 in 2003.
Executive producers: Judith Bunting and Phil Dolling
Series producer: Rachel Evans

Published by BBC Books, BBC Worldwide Ltd,
Woodlands, 80 Wood Lane, London W12 0TT

First published 2004
Text © John Marsden and Alison Dillon 2004
The moral right of the authors has been asserted.

ISBN 0 563 52136 8

Commissioning editor: Emma Shackleton
Project editor: Sarah Miles
Copy editor: Polly Boyd
Art director: Annette Peppis
Design: Grade Design Consultants, London
Picture researcher: Claire Parker
Production controller: Kenneth McKay

Set in Helvetica Neue
Printed and bound in France by Imprimerie Pollina s.a. : L93176
Colour separations by Radstock Reproductions Ltd,
Midsomer Norton

For more information about this and other BBC books,
please visit our website on www.bbcshop.com or
telephone 08700 777001.

Contents

Introduction   6

1   Eating & Drinking   10

2   The Truth About Diets   32

3   Highs & Lows   50

4   Taking Time Out   70

5   Looking Good   90

6   Love, Sex & Making Babies   110

7   Avoiding Illness   126

8   Ten Top Tips For Living Well   150

Useful Information   166

Index   174

Acknowledgements   176

Picture Credits   176

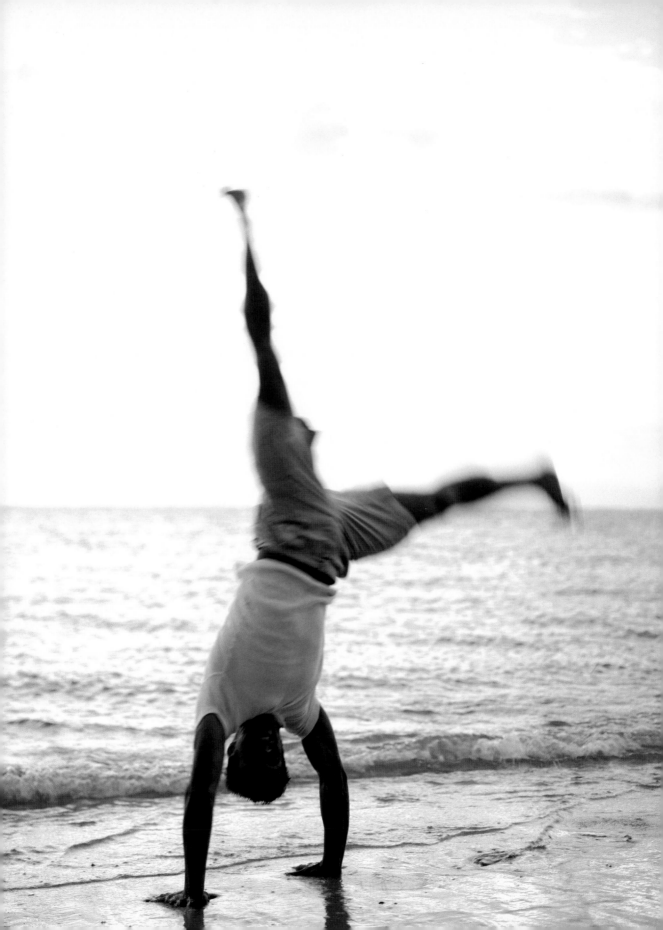

Introduction

Your body is a miraculous pleasure-seeking machine. Deep inside your brain, there are nerve pathways and chemicals that exist for the sole reason of letting you know precisely when anything you're eating, drinking, thinking or feeling is pleasurable. Scientists believe that this reaction gradually evolved thousands of years ago so that our ancestors would keep on doing all the things that were vital to their survival, such as seeking out food, water or a mate to reproduce with. It is hardly surprising, therefore, that nowadays our bodies and minds are instinctive fans of as many delicious meals, fine bottles of wine and thrillingly sensual encounters as we can muster. However, while having a hard-wired capacity to experience and enjoy life's pleasures is at the very core of being human, it also has a rather frustrating downside. You only have to take a glance at the vast number of people struggling with their weight or a substance addiction, or even the rising surge of those with symptoms of a sexually transmitted infection, to know that when it comes to pleasure, it really is possible to have too much of a good thing.

Unless you've existed in a media-free zone for the last few decades, you're bound to know that the way we choose to lead our lives will impact on the health and wellbeing of our bodies and minds. The anxiety and guilt that this fact engenders makes fertile ground for some of the very extreme and unrealistic solutions suggested for changing your lifestyle to enhance your health. In our view, extreme lifestyle changes don't work. Let's take the concept of the fad weight-loss diet, for instance. OK, so you may just about survive on carrot juice for three days and may even learn to revel in the headache-infused experience of 'de-toxing', but in the long run, this sort of plan will never make a jot of difference to your overall health for one profound reason: it is unsustainable. You simply cannot live like that for any length of time.

This book is different. We feel very strongly that you can make far less extreme changes to your lifestyle and, as a result, experience true health and wellbeing benefits. This is largely because the kind of changes we believe in don't require much time, money or effort, so they'll fit into most people's lives with ease and have real staying power. In our opinion, you don't need to worry about regular infusions of wheatgrass juice, stick puritanically to strictly macrobiotic food, consume gag-inducing detoxing herbal concoctions or have a personal trainer. In the real world, being healthy and staying that way is simply down to knowing what different lifestyle choices mean for your mind and body, and using that knowledge to shape your own life into one of vitality, good health and wellbeing in the long term.

Live Well…Be Healthy has been designed as a multipurpose book. Reading it from start to finish, you'll get an in-depth comprehensive view of how your own individual lifestyle is impacting on your health and how you can improve it through a wealth of simple and realistic measures. You'll get the low-down on topics ranging from vital everyday functions, such as eating, drinking and sleeping, through more personal areas, such as body image and emotional wellbeing, to life's milestones, such as falling in love and trying for a baby. Each chapter has also been written as a stand-alone guide to its particular topic, so that you can dip into the book to find information, advice and support on a specific problem. Chapter 7 contains individual guides to a range of illnesses for those particularly interested in preventative lifestyle choices and Chapter 8 offers our top ten tips for healthy living, for those in search of a concise yet overall guide to maximizing health and wellbeing.

This book is not about quick fixes or fads, it's about choosing good health as a way of life. We very much hope that *Live Well…Be Healthy* will throw new light on the fact that healthy living doesn't have to be complicated, restrictive or dull, but is instead a lifestyle in itself – one which you can enjoy, savour and sustain for many years to come.

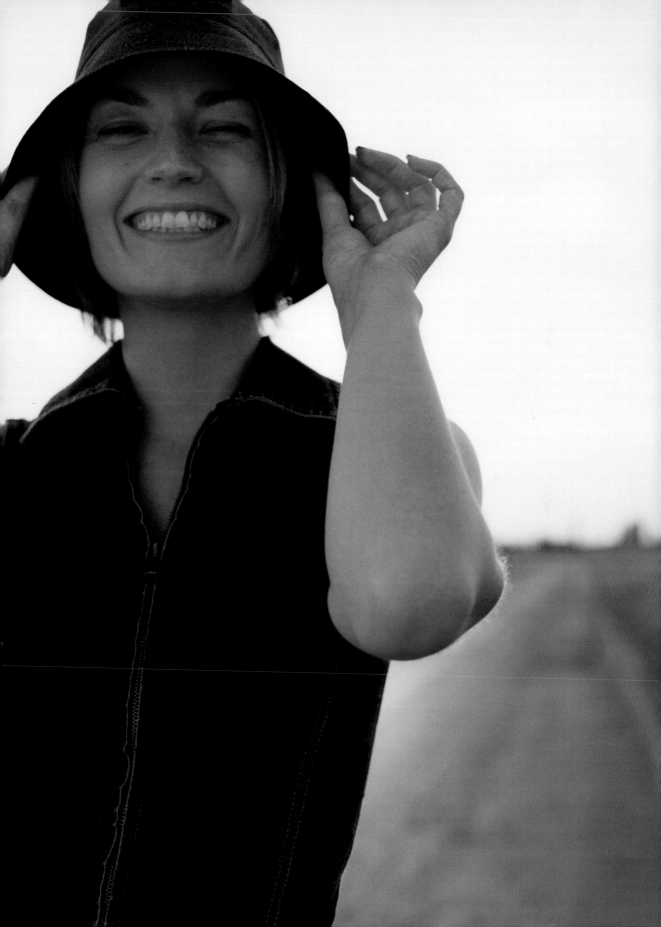

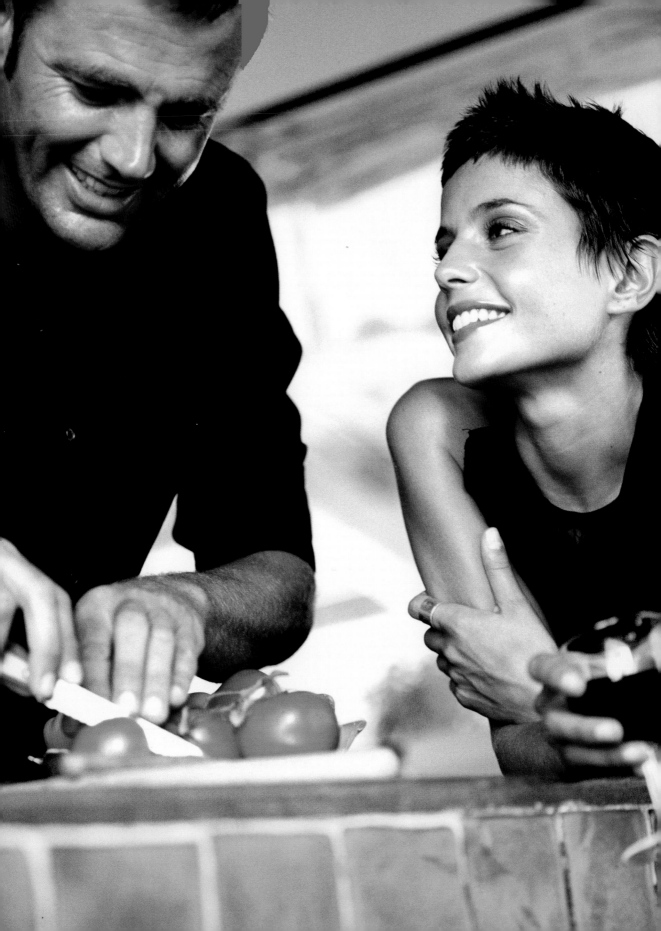

1

Eating & Drinking

No matter who you are or where you live, the very fact that you're alive depends on you eating and drinking every day. Because food and drink are so vital to our survival and success as a species, the human brain evolved a pleasure response to it. There would have been dire consequences if our ancestors had simply got bored with food and couldn't be bothered to hunt for it any more. So a combination of hunger signals and the pleasure we take in eating and drinking spurred us on through the generations to seek out food and drink. Even the sight and smell of food can trigger the release of a pleasurable and rewarding chemical called dopamine in your brain.

But while a favourite meal and a fine bottle of wine might count as one of the most satisfying sensory experiences in your life, food and drink are also directly responsible for some of our greatest health problems. Between eating to live and living to eat there lies a maze of complex and confusing factors that we must all navigate our way through to get the best from our daily diet. In this chapter we hope to help you reach a new understanding of eating and drinking healthily by laying out the facts about what your body really needs and why. We believe it's the key to unlocking the door of good health.

We'll focus on meals, drinks and even vitamin and mineral supplements and show you how understanding the basics can do wonders for your health. But don't despair too much about strict rules – eating and drinking really are two of life's greatest pleasures and we certainly don't want to be killjoys. In fact, in this chapter we'll show you how having a little bit of what you fancy can indeed do your health a lot of good.

Food for thought

If you're the kind of person who thinks of your daily diet as breakfast, lunch, dinner and a few snacks in between, then think again. The key to eating healthily is understanding the building blocks of food you eat across the whole day. While you probably see terms like 'protein' and 'carbohydrates' on food labels and in diet books and newspaper articles, do you really know what they mean to your body?

Ultimately, just as a car needs fuel to run properly, your body needs energy. In fact, the basic housekeeping uses up quite a bit – this consists of the everyday functions your body quietly gets on with, such as maintaining the health of the billions of cells that make up your body, keeping your tissues and organs working properly and making sure all the

chemical and hormonal processes going on inside you run smoothly. Once you factor in all the additional activities of work and play you get up to each day, it's clear to see why your body is so hungry for energy.

We measure energy in food by calories, also known as kilocalories, and that golden figure – which so many of us scamper to check on food labels – depends on precisely how much protein, fat and carbohydrate a food contains. There are nine calories for each gram of fat in a food and four calories for each gram of carbohydrate or protein. If the

Below: Eating a diet high in saturated fat means the level of cholesterol (shown here in yellow) in your body rises, restricting blood flow and increasing your risk of heart disease and strokes.

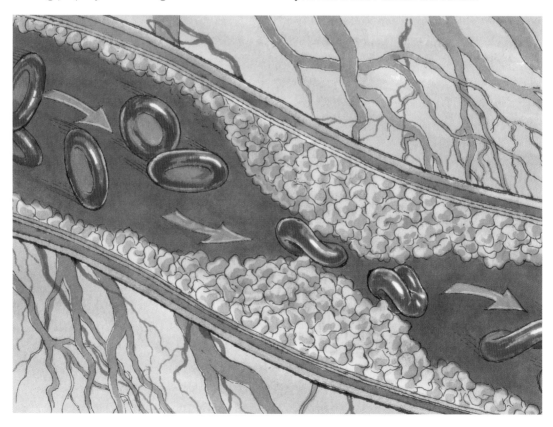

numbers are baffling you already, let's get back to basics. Here's a simple explanation of what the components of your food really are:

Protein is a nutrient found in meat, fish, eggs, pulses and nuts and is used by your body to power muscles, tendons and to keep cells working properly. It contains less than half the number of calories contained in fat, especially if you choose lean forms of protein, for example white fish or chicken with the skin removed. The method of cooking is also important – low-fat processes, such as grilling, griddling or boiling, will ensure you eat less fat than if you fry (which involves using a considerable amount of fat when you prepare the food).

Fats, contrary to popular belief, aren't all bad. In fact, they have an important part to play in healthy eating: they help transport the vitamins A, D and E to where they're needed in your body and they also keep your skin, hair and nails healthy. Fat in food also makes you feel full for longer – that's because it takes more time to digest than carbohydrates or protein. You'll find fats in cream, butter, cooking oils and all processed foods, such as sausages, crisps, pies, cakes and biscuits. Processed foods have the highest number of calories of all foods. However, some fats are better for your health than others so it's worth understanding the difference. There are three different types of 'natural' fat: saturated, monounsaturated and polyunsaturated. It's the first type you've got to watch out for. Too much saturated fat will cause your body to produce cholesterol, which builds up in your blood vessels causing heart disease and strokes. Be aware that animal fats, such as those found in dairy products, and cheaper fats used in processed food, tend to be very

high in saturated fat. Monounsaturated fats, such as olive oil, or polyunsaturated fats, such as sunflower oil, won't hike up your cholesterol levels, but bear in mind that they still contain the same high level of calories as saturated fat. Processed food manufacturers also use fats that can be chemically altered, to add value to their products. For example, liquid vegetable oils can be chemically altered to turn them into hydrogenated fats (or trans fats), which add texture to food as well as their fatty taste. Both cheap saturated fats and molecularly altered fats are particularly bad for our bodies and raise cholesterol levels substantially. As a result, many nutritionists believe that trans fats are even worse for us than saturated fats.

Carbohydrates are essentially sugars but they come in two varieties. Simple sugars, such as fructose (from fruit), lactose (from milk), glucose and sucrose (sugar as we know it), are easy for your body to absorb and use quickly, whereas carbohydrates (known as complex carbohydrates or starches), such as bread, pasta, rice, potatoes and cereal grains, are more difficult for your body to digest. As you were enjoying the very first mouthful of your breakfast cereal or croissant this morning, your pancreas, a solid gland that sits behind your stomach and measures about 25 centimetres (10 inches) long, was leaping into action. It began pumping out the hormone insulin, which serves a very important function in your body. Insulin keeps the amount of sugar in your blood in check and helps to convert it into fat stores if there's too much of it swimming around your body. Importantly, the simple sugars will cause a huge surge in insulin when you eat them, while the starches, those more complicated carbohydrates, will trigger

Ten steps to healthy meals

1 Try to eat a good mix of protein, carbohydrate and fat at every meal. If it helps to work out proportions, imagine your plate divided into percentages to be sure you're eating the right amount of each food type.

2 Always choose lean types of protein and where possible cut the fat and skin off meat, chicken and fish. Remember grilling, griddling and boiling are much better for you than frying or roasting.

3 Protein has a longer hunger-satisfying effect so rather than reaching for carbohydrates when you fancy a snack, try a few slices of low-fat cheese or a handful of nuts.

4 Try to avoid processed foods wherever possible. Although they're an economical option both in terms of time and money, you'll be eating more calories, more saturated fat and, in most cases, more salt.

5 You should aim to eat only 6 g (¼ oz) of salt a day (most of us eat around 9 g/⅓ oz). Eating too much salt tends to increase your blood pressure, which in turn puts you at risk of a stroke. Watch out for scarily high levels of salt hidden in ready meals and all processed food. Use more herbs and spices than salt when cooking, buy low-sodium salt for the table and get out of the habit of adding salt to your dinner before you've even tasted it.

6 Eat plenty of fibre – that's roughage from wholemeal bread, wholewheat pasta and brown rice, pulses, high-fibre cereals, fruits and vegetables. A diet rich in fibre means good bowel health and has been shown to be vital in preventing colon cancer.

7 As a general rule, try to eat at least five portions of different fruit or vegetables a day to ward off heart disease and many types of cancer. If you're not a fan, bear in mind that tinned vegetables and dried fruit count too.

8 Switch to using olive oil for cooking rather than butter or vegetable oil. You could also try buying a spray-oil container, which means you'll use much less. Try to use olive-oil spreads for toast and sandwiches – these tend to be better for you than butter or margarine. Regardless of your age, pay particular attention to lowering your saturated fat intake if anyone in your family suffers from heart disease or high cholesterol levels.

9 Always try to eat complex carbohydrates, such as wholemeal bread, wholewheat pasta, brown rice and wholegrain cereals, rather than refined ones. This will ensure a good steady rise in blood sugar, which means more energy for longer. If you do want to eat processed carbohydrates, such as white bread, pastries or pasta, it's better to do this earlier in the day. If you eat a huge bowl of pasta just before bed, when you're about to be entirely sedentary for several hours, there will be a lot of excess blood sugar for your insulin to convert to stored fat.

10 If you're eating out, bear in mind that the cheapest and easiest way for a restaurant to add flavour and taste to food is to add fat. Restaurant meals are likely to be much more calorific than home-cooked ones, so choose carefully – grilled meat or fish, salad and vegetables are always a good low-fat choice and fit in with the low-carbohydrate evening plan too (see tip 9).

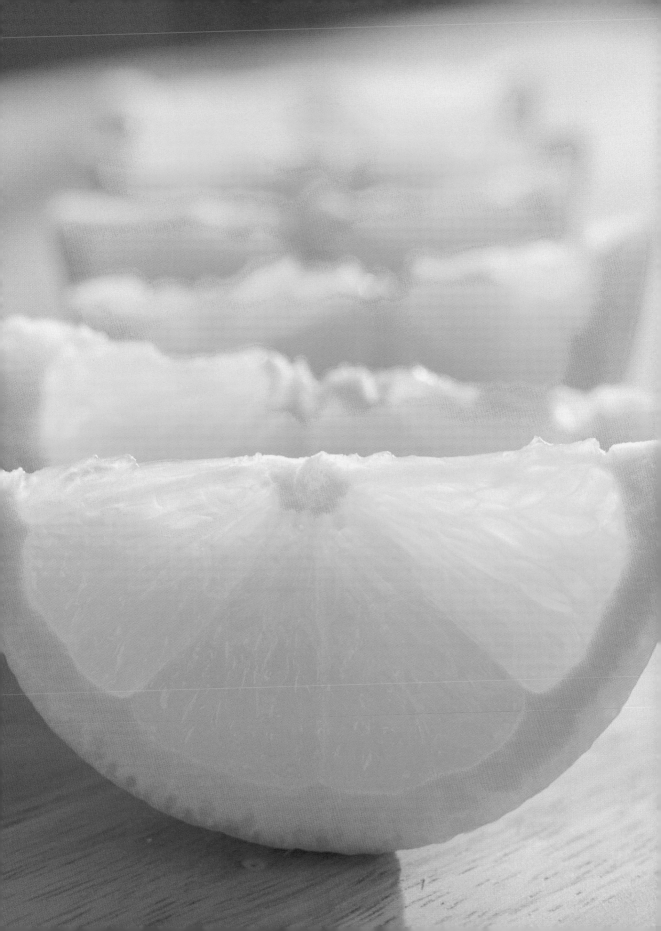

Label fable

Just because you're not watching your weight, it doesn't mean you don't need to know precisely what you're putting into your body. Packaged food is not always what it seems – food companies need to make profits and our interest in healthy eating can sometimes be a good way for them to cash in. Take our label test to find out whether you'd be fooled by the tricks of the trade.

a If I buy an item labelled as 'low fat' or 'reduced fat' it will mean I'm consuming fewer calories and will help my health overall.
TRUE/FALSE

b A food label says it has 'no artificial sweeteners' or 'no added sugar' so it must be low calorie because it's sugar-free.
TRUE/FALSE

c It's a legal requirement to include the word 'sugar' in the ingredients list if it's one of the food's ingredients.
TRUE/FALSE

d I can't be sure whether it's a healthy food or not because there's no nutritional information on the packet, only an ingredients list.
TRUE/FALSE

e I don't tend to look at the figures. As long as the packaging mentions it's a healthy option, I figure it must be OK for me to eat it.
TRUE/FALSE

Now check out how you fared:

a FALSE. This is one of the biggest mistakes you can make when shopping. While one version of a food item can have lower fat than another, that doesn't necessarily mean that it has fewer calories. Take a look at the fat and carbohydrate figures of a full-fat and low-fat yoghurt. The fact is, if you take fat out you need to substitute something else to make up for the loss of flavour. In most cases, manufacturers add sugar to replace fat, which means that when it comes to hiking up your blood-sugar levels, some low-fat products aren't as healthy as you think.

b FALSE. Sugar or artificial sweeteners may not have been added, but the food itself may contain naturally occurring sugars, such as fructose (from fruit) or lactose (from milk). Your body can't tell the difference between natural and artificial sugars.

c FALSE. It is a legal requirement to list all ingredients but when you're watching out for sugar, bear in mind you'll also need to take stock of any labels quoting glucose, invert sugar, sucrose, dextrose, honey, treacle, golden syrup, maple syrup, hydrolyzed starch or even fruit juice concentrate.

d FALSE. It's not ideal to rely on an ingredients list alone, but do remember that the higher up the list an ingredient comes, the more of it there is in the product.

e FALSE. Avoid relying on generalizations like 'healthy option'. To be certain, you need to know the calorie content per serving.

a slower, gentler rise of the hormone. In other words, it's best to ensure that the majority of your carbohydrate intake is made up of starchy foods; don't overdo the simple sugars. Do bear in mind, however, that processed or refined carbohydrates, for example white bread, rice and pasta, contain much higher amounts of simple sugars than wholegrain versions do, so opt for brown rice, wholewheat pasta, wholemeal bread and wholegrain cereals whenever possible.

How much is enough?

Knowing whether a food contains protein, carbohydrate or fat is only half the battle – it's also vital you know how much of each you need every day. The truth is that the actual amount of energy and nutrients you need from food varies enormously depending on factors like your age, sex and genetic make-up. Your metabolism is the unique rate at which your body burns up the calories you've consumed. The younger you are, the faster this will occur as there will be a greater number of cells growing and dividing in your body. The taller and heavier you are, the faster your metabolism will be – so women lose out in that arena as men have a greater percentage of heavier muscle tissue than fat in their bodies. If you live in a tropical or extremely cold environment, your calorie-burning rate could be up to 20 per cent higher as a result. And as we all know, regular exercise also increases your metabolic rate.

When it comes to working out how much food you need to keep your body running properly, you should follow some simple rules. If you're generally happy with your weight and you're a man you need to eat around 2500 calories a day. For a woman to maintain her weight she'll need around 1900 calories a day. (We'll be looking at calorie requirements for those not so content with their weight in Chapter 2.) But of those 1900 or 2500 calories you need to consume each day, how much should be fat, carbohydrate or protein?

It's very important that fats (especially the less healthy saturated ones) shouldn't exceed more than 30 per cent of your daily diet. Nutritionists suggest that around 25 per cent of your food should be made up of protein with the remaining 45 per cent being carbohydrates, fruit and vegetables. For the last 25 years, governments around the western world have recommended that we eat carbohydrates as our basic staple food, which we then supplement with a smaller amount of protein, and even less fat. In recent years, there has been much controversy over whether such a high-carb eating plan actually leads to good health. Critics have linked high consumption of carbohydrates with a massive rise in the number of overweight and obese people around the world. The enormous success of low-carb and even no-carb slimming diets has caught everyone's eye and we'll be exploring these in the following chapter. However, the key point to remember here is that for healthy nutrition you always need to think about balance. Your body needs carbohydrates for good health, just as it needs protein and fats. Follow our simple tips and advice on how you can make food work for you (see page 14).

Pill power

You probably know that vitamins and minerals play an important part in keeping your body working healthily, but let's get to the bottom of whether you really need any extra ones. A recent survey showed that almost 50 per cent of the American population now feels the need to supplement their food intake with vitamin or mineral pills, and thousands of tablets are sold across the world every day.

You do need to be aware that the all-round reputation of supplements as being 'natural' doesn't necessarily mean they're always good for your health – deadly nightshade, hemlock and arsenic are all natural too and you certainly wouldn't choose to pop any of them in pill form. You must also bear in mind that while supplements do have effects on your body, most have never been clinically tested or checked (it's not yet a legal requirement although regulations around the world are improving). In some cases, scientists don't even know whether exceeding the suggested dose could have life-threatening effects on your body.

The fact is that if you regularly eat a good balanced diet, you should be getting all your body's required vitamins and minerals from your food. But of course there are plenty of reasons why that could not be the case: you may have recently been very stressed, busy at work, travelling abroad or suffering from an illness. You might be a very strict vegetarian or on a low-calorie weight-loss diet. When you feel run-down and turn to a health store for a supplement pick-me-up, what's the safest way to go about it? Follow our checklist (see opposite).

Live a little

It's not just the food you choose to eat that can affect your health – how you feel about it can also take its toll, especially if you're concerned about your weight or body image. To keep your eating healthy in body and mind, follow our five key principles for long-lasting food wellbeing:

Be sensible. Think about your personal metabolism, based not only on your age,

sex, body size, lifestyle and genetic make-up, but also on a day-by-day basis. If you're exercising that day, you can afford to eat a little more, whereas if you're having a very sedentary time at work or home, try to cut back a little. It's not rocket science, but it does mean you can vary your diet somewhat without feeling guilty.

Good or bad? Try not to think about food in terms of it being good or bad. No single food can be 'bad' for you on its own, nor can any one food be 'good' for you in isolation. This way of thinking will take its toll on your self-esteem and how you see yourself. There will be days when you want to eat foods you might class as bad, but punishing yourself about it afterwards won't help your overall wellbeing. If you occasionally eat something you consider to be unhealthy, enjoy it but then make sure it's a special treat that you balance out with regular periods of healthy eating and exercise at other times.

Listen to your body. As children, most of us were praised for leaving an empty plate at the dinner table. We tend to eat until our portion is finished, but that's not always what your body wants. Try two tests. First, when it comes round to lunchtime tomorrow, take a moment to think about whether you actually do feel physically hungry before you get going on that sandwich. If not, wait a bit longer until you really do feel the hunger set in. You may find that your body is better suited to five small meals through the day, rather than three large ones at set meal times. Also when you sit down for your next meal, try eating more slowly than usual and see if you can identify when your body feels physically full. By relying more on your body's signals of hunger and satiety, you'll naturally

Supplement checklist

• When the need for supplements strikes, try buying a comprehensive one-a-day multivitamin and mineral tablet from a reputable health store. This should help your body make up for recent vitamin and mineral losses and will provide safe amounts within recommended guidelines.

• Wherever possible, try then to adjust your diet to get more nutrients. It is always healthier to get vitamins and minerals from foods than from a pill. Don't just reach for a pill when you can boost vitamin and mineral levels through fresh food.

• If you decide to buy a single supplement pill, be careful about sticking to the RDA (recommended daily amount) or RDV (recommended daily value), unless you're advised otherwise by a medical doctor. More doesn't always mean better; even simple supplements like vitamin A and vitamin D can be dangerous if taken in large amounts.

• Don't use supplements as a way of self-medicating. If you are suffering symptoms like chronic tiredness, lack of energy, paleness, weakness or pain of any description, it's always best to get them checked out by a doctor.

• Be aware that if you are taking any other medication it could interact with over-the-counter supplements. For instance, St John's Wort can help people suffering from mild depression but it can also reduce the effectiveness of the contraceptive pill. Calcium supplements can affect the way that antibiotics are absorbed. It's always best to check with your doctor or pharmacist before starting supplements.

• If you are a vegetarian or have heavy periods, you should consider taking an iron supplement in addition to a general multivitamin.

• You should take a separate supplement of folic acid if you are pregnant or considering having a baby soon. Studies have shown that it significantly reduces the chances of your baby being born with a neural tube defect, such as spina bifida. It is most important to take it in the first three months of pregnancy. Unless you're advised to do so by a doctor or midwife, don't take other supplements during pregnancy as they could have harmful effects on your growing baby.

• If you are put on a course of antibiotics, they're likely to wipe out the good bacteria in your gut as well as the bad bacteria they were prescribed for. You could consider taking a probiotic supplement, such as acidophilus, until the course of medicines is complete.

• Research has shown that omega-3 oils, found in oily fish such as fresh tuna, trout, anchovies, sardines, pilchards, kippers and herring, can boost your circulation and protect the health of your heart and brain. If you don't eat oily fish regularly, consider taking a daily fish oil supplement to make sure you get the beneficial health effects of omega-3 oils.

• Try not to get obsessed about supplement levels. Becoming overly concerned about any aspect of diet and nutrition can lead to anxiety, stress and eating disorders.

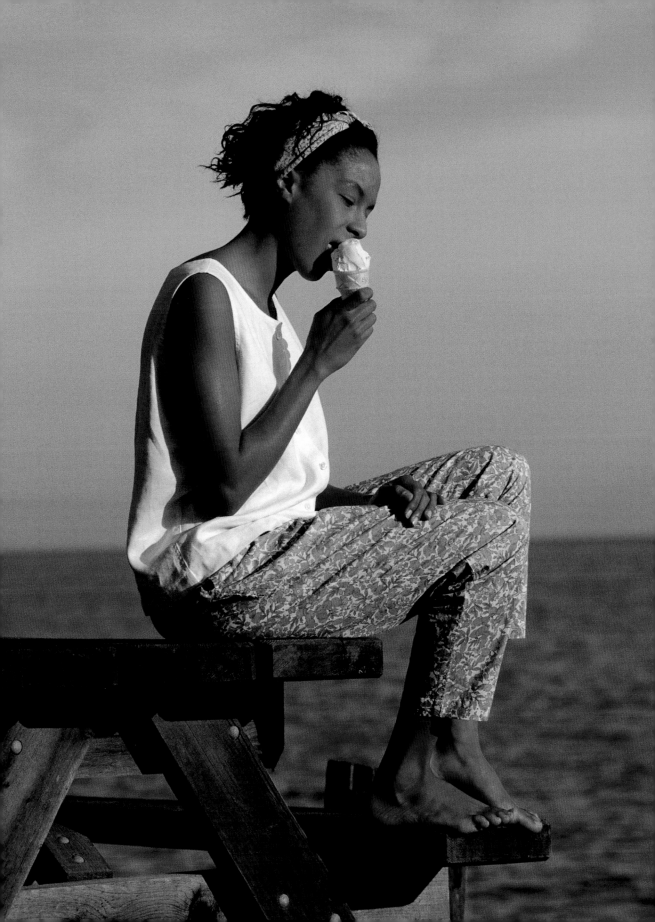

adjust your food intake to match your physiological needs much better.

Constant craving. Unfortunately, hunger isn't always what it seems. Because food is so intricately intertwined with feelings of pleasure, we can crave it for all sorts of reasons other than needing nutrients. Amazingly, scientists in the US have recently found that fat and sugar seem to put a brake on the chemical reaction that's going on in the body when we're stressed, which could explain why some of us reach for unhealthy comfort foods when the going gets tough. If you find yourself regularly eating more than you think your body needs, make a mental checklist of other reasons why you might be eating. It could be times when you're angry, sad, hurt or simply bored. By identifying the possibilities, you'll be one big step towards getting your eating back on a healthy track.

Enjoy food. There's even a name now for being obsessed with healthy eating – orthorexia. Ironically, taking healthy eating to its extreme can leave you with some of the same obsessive compulsive symptoms as people suffering from eating disorders. Increasing numbers of people claim to be intolerant to certain food groups, such as wheat or dairy, and give these foods up altogether. In fact, only two per cent of the population are officially allergic to wheat or dairy. Unless you have a medically proven allergy to foods like these, beware of giving up whole food groups. Without any dairy products your body will miss out on vital calcium supplies, and by cutting out wheat entirely you could be losing one of your main fibre sources, putting you at

Left: Be informed about what you're eating, but treat yourself from time to time – life's too short not to!

high risk of poor bowel health. If you're suffering from symptoms you believe are related to a food allergy or intolerance, get them properly checked out by your doctor. Being extremely strict and rigid with your diet and what you feel is healthy is never good for your physical or emotional wellbeing. The occasional pizza, chocolate cake or bottle of red wine are there to be enjoyed as special food treats. Indulging yourself now and again is one of the joys of life!

Let's have a drink

Alcohol is so closely woven into the fabric of our lives that even the simple invitation to 'have a drink' suggests an alcoholic tipple to most of us. Drinking is so commonplace that few of us stop to think that we're taking a drug at all. But, in fact, alcohol is the world's oldest mood-altering drug. Our ancestors had their first contact with it when they ate very ripe fruits that had naturally fermented (the basis for making wine) and knowledge about brewing and distilling beer and spirits using cereals has been in place for thousands of years.

Today, nine out of ten people in the UK drink alcohol on a regular basis. Most people enjoy socializing with friends over a few drinks – it's one of our nation's favourite pastimes. Drinking makes us feel more relaxed, less inhibited, more talkative and our everyday worries seem to fade away. Having said that, many people do seem to like the effects of alcohol a bit too much; it's important to remember that alcohol is a potent sedative drug, capable of causing us serious harm if we overdo it. Every year in the UK, 20,000 people get up to mischief when drinking and get arrested; 13,000 get into drunken fights and 600 people are murdered while either they or their attacker are intoxicated. And those are just the immediate consequences of excessive boozing. So, if you enjoy a drink or two, the trick is to make sure you get all the benefits without suffering the downsides – and that means learning to manage your alcohol intake safely and healthily.

What's in your glass?

Because different types of alcoholic drinks and the various brands vary in their strength, it's a good idea to know how much alcohol is inside that bottle or can. By law, all drinks have an indication of this stated on the packaging. You should look for the alcohol by volume percentage, or % AbV. Scanning for AbV information is useful but it isn't a particularly helpful way of keeping an eye on your actual drinking. Instead, it's much easier to know about the number of standard units of alcohol that are in your pint, glass or short.

As it happens, one standard unit contains 10 ml (just under ½ fl oz) of pure alcohol and this is approximately equal to half a pint of ordinary strength beer; one pub glass of wine or a single shot of spirits. It's useful to know that the AbV also indicates the number of units in 1 litre (1¾ pints) of a drink. So, a litre of 12 per cent AbV wine has…12 units! Below you'll find a table of typical drinks, showing their AbV content, the number of units they contain and the number of calories this represents (for the record, there's about 5.5 calories in every millilitre of pure alcohol).

Remember, this table is just a rough guide. There are some drinks that pack a truly phenomenal punch. The spirit drink absinthe, for example, is about 68 per cent AbV and then there's the vast range of cocktails: a margarita contains a double shot of tequila and a shot of Cointreau (4.2 units a pop). Pure alcohol itself has no nutritional value but, as the table shows, it does contain energy in the form of simple sugars – which means you can notch up quite a few liquid calories if you're not careful.

Drink	% AbV	Units	Calories
Pint standard beer/lager (568 ml)	3.5–4.5	2.0–2.5	109–41
Pint strong beer/lager	5–6	2.5–3.4	156–87
Pint cider	6–8	3.4–4.5	187–250
Bottle of 'alcopop' (330 ml)	5–5.5	1.7–1.8	91–100
Standard glass of wine (125 ml)	12–14	1.5–1.8	83–96
Large glass of wine (175 ml)	12–14	2.1–2.5	116–35
Bottle of wine (75 cl)	12–14	9.0–10.5	495–578
Single measure of spirits (35 ml)	38–40	1.3–1.4	73–77

How alcohol goes to work

The precise effects of alcohol depend on lots of different factors including the type of drink, how strong it is, how quickly you gulp it down, your body weight and constitution, the amount of food in your stomach, other medicines or drugs you may have taken and even your emotional state.

As you drain your glass, alcohol gets steadily absorbed in your stomach and within five to ten minutes reaches your bloodstream. It then enters and dissolves into the water inside each tissue in your body, with the exception of fat tissue (alcohol can't dissolve into fat). About 5 per cent of the alcohol in your drink is removed from the body by the lungs (which is why the amount you've drunk can be estimated by a Breathalyzer) and your kidneys get rid of another 5 per cent. The remaining 90 per cent is handled directly by your liver.

By the time alcohol reaches the tissues in the body, you'll start to feel its effects. But how powerful those effects are will depend on your blood alcohol concentration or BAC. The BAC is the amount of alcohol that is found in 100 ml (3½ fl oz) of blood expressed as a percentage and it's a good indicator of the amount of alcohol in the body. As a very general rule, one unit of alcohol raises a man's BAC within the first hour by 0.02 per cent and a woman's by 0.03 per cent.

What drink does to you

Let's follow the stages of how alcohol takes effect on your mind and body. After the first few drinks, you'll be relaxed and euphoric, with a BAC of between 0.02 and 0.12 per cent. You'll probably feel more relaxed and confident, talkative and daring, but bear in mind that alcohol is actually a sedative drug –

Case Study
Weekday booze control

Leoni, 26, found that drinking had become a very central part of her working week. 'I work in a busy, lively office and we're always having a laugh. A year ago, I got into the habit of going to the pub across the street after work with some friends from work.' While she really enjoyed this as a way to unwind, Leoni rarely left without having five drinks and she was shocked to realize that after taking her big night out on the town on Saturday into account, her weekly drinks total was up to 30 units. 'I'd started to feel really awful in the mornings and my work was beginning to suffer a bit: I'd been late four or five times and just hadn't felt as sharp as I used to.' During a test for a new medical insurance policy she completed a drink diary and talked about her drinking with the doctor. 'I realized that part of the problem was that I would go to the pub after work with five friends and we'd each get a round; so I'd always have five drinks. So I dropped out of most of the pub sessions but when I did go, I reduced my drinks to three, kicking off with a non-alcoholic first drink and buying myself a lime and soda when it was my round.' With a bit of further restraint at the weekend, Leoni had turned around her drinking total and got her units down to a total of 16 for the week. 'I really haven't found it difficult at all: I still go out and have fun, and it's so much better to wake up feeling clear-headed. I've also really enjoyed having a bit of extra money now that my drinks bill is lower.'

Battle of the sexes: dealing with drink

● Women are more affected by alcohol than men. There are three reasons why: the first is body weight – the fact that women are generally lighter than men means that there's less body mass to absorb it; but the second and more important factor is the water content of the body – women have a lower body water content than men, so if a woman and a man drink together, drink for drink, the woman's blood alcohol concentration will be up to 50 per cent higher than the man's. The third factor is that men have more of an enzyme called alcohol dehydrogenase in their stomachs. This enzyme assists the liver in breaking down alcohol, so men absorb less alcohol into their bloodstream than women.

● But it's not all good news for men either. The long-term effects of drinking can take a serious toll on the male physique. Over time, alcohol reduces a man's level of the natural sex hormone testosterone and increases the very small levels of oestrogen circulating around his body. Long-term heavy alcohol use can even lead to a condition in which a man's breast tissue can become feminized – a condition called gynaecomastia (as the illustration below shows).

● In women, alcohol works in the reverse way on the sex hormones. It increases the very tiny, naturally produced levels of the male sex hormone testosterone and in very

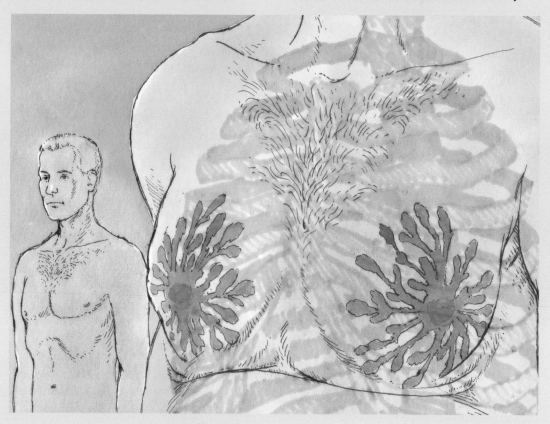

heavy-drinking females that can mean masculinizing effects such as more body and facial hair and even a deeper voice.

● Scientists have shown that around 60 per cent of women who consume eight standard drinks a day (which amounts to 120 ml/4 fl oz of pure alcohol) suffer from delayed ovulation or even no ovulation at all.

● Men who are heavy long-term drinkers can also damage their testicles and sperm. Alcohol seems to have an effect on the seminiferous tubules in a man's testicles by decreasing their diameter. It also causes some local scarring and general contraction of the testicles themselves. On top of that, the sperm themselves can reduce in number and also fail to develop properly.

Left: Heavy drinking over many years can cause levels of the female sex hormone oestrogen to increase significantly in some men, causing the tissue in the chest area to develop into a more female 'breast-like' shape.

so you'll already be less mentally alert and your memory and concentration will start to be affected.

In the second stage of intoxication, your BAC will be between 0.13 and 0.20 per cent, drowsiness will set in, your reaction time will be diminished and your judgement and coordination will be affected. After that, you'll reach a stage of drunkenness in which you become confused and agitated. Your speech may be slurred, delicate movements would be out of the question and your emotional temperature is raised – you're likely to seriously misjudge social cues and that BAC is still rising: at this stage, you'd be between 0.21 and 0.30 per cent.

If your BAC gets as high as somewhere between 0.31 and 0.40 per cent, you'll be in a stage of intoxication known as stupor. It's serious: you're probably barely able to move and nausea and vomiting are likely. Beyond 0.40 per cent and you'll face the risk of unconsciousness. With your heart rate and respiration falling fast, a seizure or even a coma might occur. For most people, this level of BAC is enough to be a fatal dose.

While thankfully most of us never get to sample the effects of having a sky-high blood alcohol concentration, many more of us regularly get to the stage of intoxication where driving is dangerous. In the UK and in many states in the US, the current legal limit for driving is a BAC of 0.08 per cent, which equals about two and a half pints of ordinary strength beer, depending on the person, of course. As we've just described, this level would mean you were in the very first stages of intoxication. Elsewhere in Europe, the BAC limit is as low as 0.05 per cent. Most police forces use a roadside breath test as a convenient means of checking how much you've had. The best advice is to avoid drink altogether if you're driving. It's simply not worth the potentially tragic consequences. Take turns with your partner or a friend to be the designated non-drinking driver on your evenings out.

The dreaded hangover

As most of us know only too well, the dreaded hangover is a queasy mix of headache, nausea and fatigue that greets us the morning after the night before. But why does a hangover happen, and how can you cope with its effects or – more importantly – how can you avoid getting one in the first place?

Drinking alcohol has a strong diuretic effect, which means you'll discharge more liquid than you take in. Alcohol acts on the pituitary gland in the brain and stops production of a hormone called vasopressin, which tells the kidneys to reabsorb water that was heading for the bladder. In turn, the body takes water from other areas, for instance, from your brain – and this has the effect of shrinking it slightly, causing that familiar headache. While you're making frequent trips to the lavatory on your night out, you're also depleting essential

Top tips for beating hangovers

- **Eat before you drink.** A light meal is ideal before you set out for a few drinks; a carbohydrate-based meal is probably best to slow down alcohol absorption, and make sure you drink plenty of non-alcoholic fluids as well before you go out.

- **Boost your body's chances.** Some people take B complex vitamins, particularly B6 (pyridoxine), to assist the body in breaking down the alcohol in your system. Others take a vitamin supplement containing an amino acid called N-acetyl-cysteine (NAC). NAC boosts levels of a liver enzyme called glutathione, which mop up nasty chemicals called free radicals, which can build up in the liver when we drink large quantities of alcohol.

- **Rehydrate.** Drinking a lot of alcohol over the course of an evening turns on your urine flow to the max. In an ideal world, try to space out alcoholic drinks during the evening with water. If you match each tipple with a big glass of water you're likely to hardly suffer at

all the next day. But failing that, before turning in, try to drink some water (at least 250 ml/½ pint and not more than 850 ml/1½ pints or you'll feel bloated and nauseous) to help your body rehydrate as you sleep.

- **Pain management.** You might want to consider taking a soluble aspirin (assuming you're not allergic to this medicine) or an over-the-counter hangover remedy before turning in to get some pain relief on board. Alternatively, if you wake very early, have an aspirin handy by the bedside, drink some more water and try to get some more sleep.

- **The aftermath.** You may not feel like it, but having some food is a good idea; something basic like toast or a bacon sandwich will settle your stomach and give you some welcome energy. Do not consider trying 'hair of the dog': resorting to another alcoholic tipple first thing in the morning might make you feel slightly better at first, but you'll just be delaying the inevitable, so deal with it!

sodium and potassium ions, which perform an important role in supplying your muscles with energy – their loss seems to lead to headaches and nausea. And as alcohol is broken down in your body, two nasty chemicals – formaldehyde and formic acid – are released and these are also thought to contribute to the hangover headache. To round it all off, alcohol also has a nasty habit of raiding your energy stores of glycogen sugars in the liver, leaving you feeling fatigued the next day.

If you're heading for a big night out and you reckon a hangover could be on the cards, try following our tips (see opposite) to minimize the post-alcohol suffering.

The truth about long-term drinking

Long-term heavy drinking is definitely a risk factor for your health. First of all, as we've seen, alcohol is pretty calorie-rich and heavy drinkers are often overweight. Alcohol also destroys vitamin B1 (thiamine), a nutrient that is important for healthy brain functioning, so you can definitely lose brain power over time. Research has shown that in comparison with moderate drinkers or abstainers, long-term heavy drinkers have a much greater risk of weight gain, emotional and mental problems, work and stress difficulties and physical health problems including stomach cancers and diseases of the heart, liver and pancreas. The bottom line is that excessive drinkers are 12 times more likely to die of liver cirrhosis, three times more likely to die in a car accident and six times more likely to commit suicide.

Are you overdoing it?

It's worth taking time to assess your current alcohol intake. Most people find they're drinking more than they realize. First, make a quick estimate of how many units you drink across a typical week on average (see box below). How did you do? The latest weekly guidelines were set out in 1995 by the UK government as no more than 3 to 4 drinks per day for men (21 to 28 units per week) and 2 to 3 drinks for women (14 to 21 units per week), with two non-drinking days after a heavy session. It's thought that men who drink between 21 and 50 units a week and women who drink between 14 and 35 units a week are at risk of health problems. Men and women who top these limits are thought to be drinking at dangerous levels.

In the UK, about a third of men and around one in five women drink above the recommended limits – and the proportion of women drinking above the limits has gone up by 70 per cent since 1988. Knocking back twice the daily recommended amount in one session (or binge drinking) has become more common – although many people go way beyond this. Among 16 to 24 year olds in the

	Monday	Tuesday	Wednesday	Thursday	Friday	Saturday	Sunday	Total
Lunch								
Evening								
							Grand total	

Rate your relationship with alcohol

Think back over the last three months and answer these questions as truthfully as you can:

1 How often have you drunk alcohol?
Never = 0 points
Once or twice = 2 points
Monthly (1 to 3 times) = 3 points
Weekly (1 to 4 times a week) = 4 points
Almost daily (5 to 7 times a week) = 6 points
Your score ☐

2 How often have you had a strong desire to drink?
Never = 0 points
Once or twice = 3 points
Monthly (1 to 3 times) = 4 points
Weekly (1 to 4 times a week) = 5 points
Almost daily (5 to 7 times a week) = 6 points
Your score ☐

3 How often has your alcohol use led to health, social, legal or financial problems?
Never = 0 points
Once or twice = 4 points
Monthly (1 to 3 times) = 5 points
Weekly (1 to 4 times a week) = 6 points
Almost daily (5 to 7 times a week) = 7 points
Your score ☐

4 Has a friend or family member ever expressed concern about your drinking?
No, never = 0 points
Yes, but not in the past 3 months = 3 points
Yes, in the past 3 months = 6 points
Your score ☐

5 How often have you failed to do what was normally expected of you because you'd been drinking?
Never = 0 points
Once or twice = 5 points
Monthly (1 to 3 times) = 6 points
Weekly (1 to 4 times a week) = 7 points
Almost daily (5 to 7 times a week) = 8 points
Your score ☐

Now add up your scores to work out your total ☐

What your score means:
0 to 10 = Your drinking is at safe levels.

11 to 26 = It's worth making some changes and reducing your drinking (see pages 30–1 for our top ten tips for cutting down).

27 or more = You should definitely make some changes and it may be a good idea to talk to your doctor for some additional support and advice.

These questions are reproduced from a questionnaire compiled by the WHO ASSIST Working Group (2002) called *The Alcohol, Smoking and Substance Involvement Screening Test (ASSIST): development, reliability and feasibility. Addiction, 97, 1183–1194.*

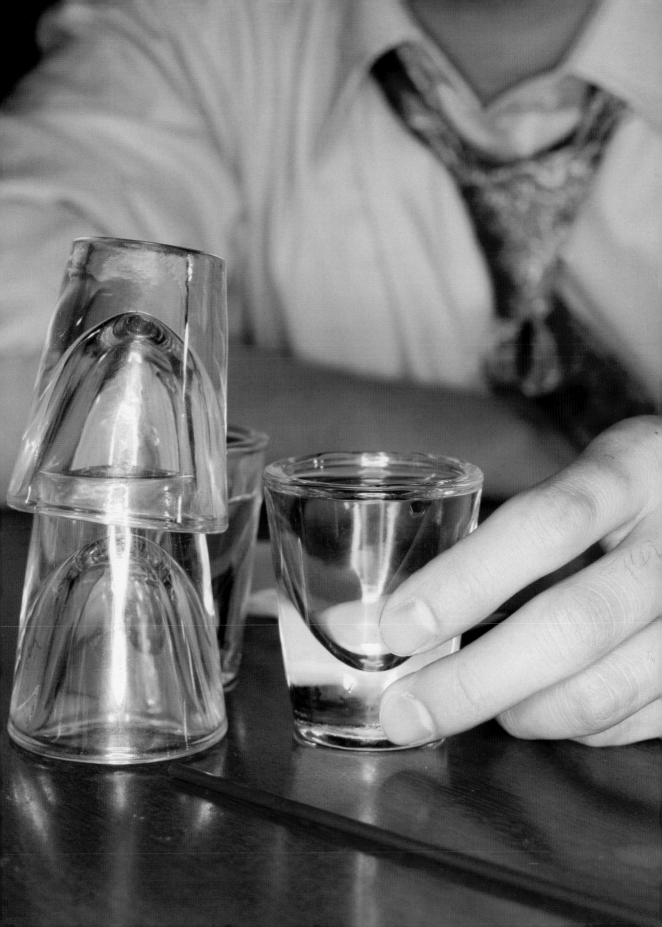

Ten top tips for cutting down

Many people decide to make changes to their drinking habits at some point and for all sorts of different reasons. Some decide that they'd like a break from a routine of regular social drinking that has begun to feel a bit stale and boring; others gradually realize that drink has started to cause a few problems at home or at work and decide to ease back a bit. If you feel the need to reduce your alcohol intake, try the following strategies:

- **Set yourself a goal.** Each person will have their own reasons for changing their drinking and will set their own goals. Be realistic; don't set a goal that you're unlikely to achieve or equally one that's unlikely to make any real difference. Think about what changes you're hoping to see – for example, sleeping better, no headaches in the morning, no more silly arguments with friends and family or even just more money in your pocket. Be clear about why you're doing this.

- **Talk to your family and friends about your decision.** There's no need to make a big deal about it, but telling those who are close to you brings your resolve into the open and you can get support and encouragement.

- **Decide which days will be 'no-drinking' days.** Your body really benefits from a good number of non-drinking days. Obviously this is down to personal preference but at least two alcohol-free days a week is a good start; and remember not to pile on the units on the remaining days!

- **Choose something to do on the non-drinking days.** What's going to replace the time you normally spend drinking? This is an opportunity to treat yourself in a new and different way – you could go to a movie, head off to the gym or have a relaxing bath at home.

- **Change your drinking style.** When you're out for a few drinks, try to quench your first thirst with a non-alcoholic drink. Soda and lime is a good choice. Also, think about how you drink – avoid gulping, drink more slowly and pace your drinking, add soda to white wine, change to weaker brands and avoid drinking shorts at the end of an evening. That 'one for the road' is never a good idea.

- **Watch out for high-risk drinking situations.** Are there certain situations that seem to lead to lots of drinking? Think about when you drink (it might mostly occur after a stressful day or on a Friday night) and what sort of company you're with when it happens. When those situations arise, prepare yourself mentally in advance to manage them better without the need for a drink.

- **Set limits.** You need to set some sensible drinking limits. Know the AbV strength of what you're drinking and avoid exceeding a set number of units (see page 22). You may want to keep a drink diary for a while so you can record how much you're drinking and monitor your progress (see page 27).

- **Learn to deal with little slips.** Most people who change their drinking style find that in spite of their best intentions, there are times when the plan goes out of the window. If this happens, try to shrug it off – follow our hangover management guide on page 26, have two alcohol-free days, then get back to the plan again.

- **Watch out for home drinking.** Many people pour larger measures and use bigger glasses at home than in a bar or pub. And reaching for a glass of wine or a can of beer as soon as you get home isn't the best move if you're trying to cut down. Go for a non-alcoholic option until you're settled and relaxed or don't drink at all at home for a while.

- **Reward yourself for your progress.** Buy yourself something or give yourself a treat as a reward for sticking to your plan – remember, another incentive for cutting down on your drinking is more money in your pocket.

UK, 37 per cent of men and 27 per cent of women regularly drink twice the daily recommended level.

If you're pregnant you need to avoid getting drunk. Some experts recommend avoiding alcohol altogether during pregnancy, but the latest evidence suggests that drinking a couple of small glasses of ordinary strength wine (12% AbV) with food up to twice a week will not cause your baby any significant harm.

Now that you've checked out your weekly units, try filling in the short questionnaire on page 28.

Below: If you're cutting down, drink half measures when out with friends and have lots of water too.

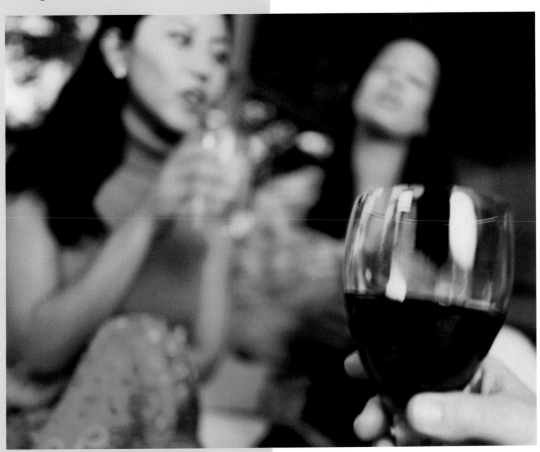

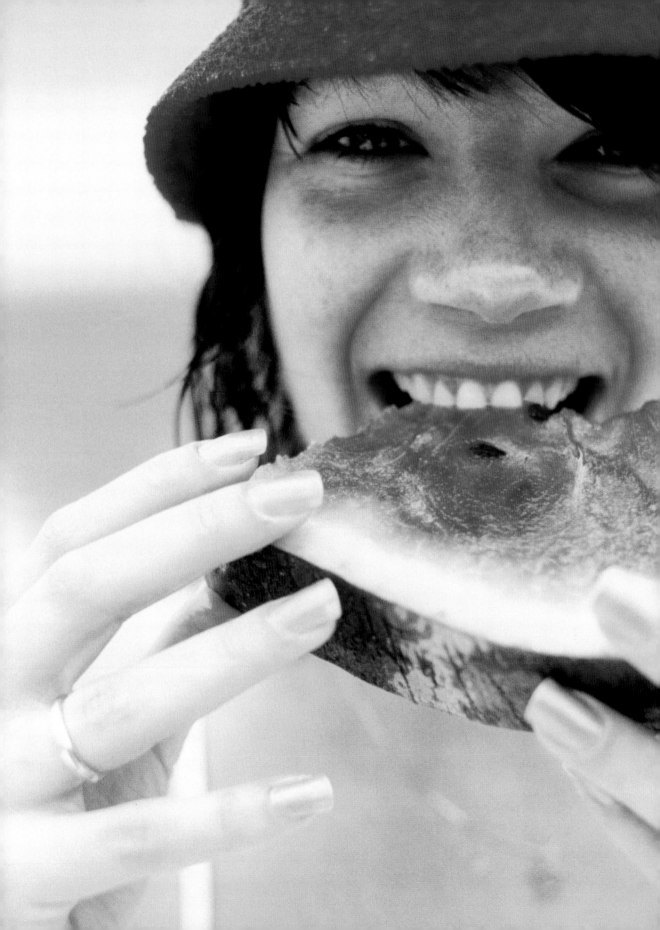

2

The Truth About Diets

It sounds simple – eat more calories than your body burns up and the excess energy will get stored as fat; eat fewer calories than you need and you'll lose weight. Yet for a staggering number of us that straightforward equation is the root of an obsession that dominates our lives. It's estimated that one billion people around the world are overweight, while 300 million of those are clinically obese. In many countries, such as the UK and US, over half the population is affected. As quickly as the figures rise, so does our desperation to achieve the perfect body and an ideal weight – in fact, the American population spends more each year on the beauty and fitness industries than on education or social services.

Now that our world is less dominated by the traditional divisions of class and money, we find ourselves more likely to be judged on our physical appearance and weight. But before you put that down to media-induced superficiality, bear in mind that being overweight or obese carries an enormous health risk. It causes more ill-health than smoking, and in the western world, an astonishing 500,000 people die every year from obesity-related diseases. Good reason, then, to lose those extra kilos. But how?

If you've ever wanted to lose weight, you'll know how easy it is to get caught up in a whirlwind of dieting. Within weeks you're back where you started, possibly having *gained* a few extra kilos. So why is losing weight so difficult? And are you aware how it's affecting your mental and emotional wellbeing? In this chapter we'll tread the rocky road of diets and detoxes to show how you can strike a balance between being a healthy weight and having a positive attitude about eating – and, in turn, feel better about yourself.

Are you a healthy weight?

First things first – it's important to know where you come on the scale of healthy weight. Grab a calculator for a rough and ready way of finding out:

● Take your height in metres and square it (multiply it by itself). Then divide your weight in kilos by this number and you have your body-mass index (BMI). For example, a woman who was 1.6 metres tall and who weighed 60 kg would have a BMI of approximately 23 (1.6 x 1.6 = 2.56, 60 ÷ 2.56 = 23.4375).

● If you prefer to work with imperial measurements, take your height in inches and square it, then divide your weight in pounds by this number and multiply the result by 703 to get your BMI.

Your BMI should fall in the range from 20 to 25. If it's less than 20 you're underweight. If it's between 25 and 30 you are overweight and if it's over 30 you are clinically obese. The BMI has been the traditional means of testing weight for some time but it's essentially quite a crude measure because it doesn't take into account the fact that lean muscle tissue is actually heavier than fat. So if your muscles are very well developed, your BMI rating could seem to indicate you are obese, even though your levels of body fat are actually quite healthy.

To get a clearer idea of whether or not your weight poses health risks, try measuring your waist circumference. Take a measuring tape around your waist over the navel. If you're a man and the measurement is greater than 102 centimetres (40 inches), you're overweight and are at risk of encountering health problems in the future as a result. For a woman, that health risk relates to waist measurements above 88 centimetres (35 inches). Finally, measure your waist-to-hip ratio by dividing your waist size by your hip circumference. If the figure is 1.0 or higher, your weight is in the danger zone for health problems. The ideal ratio for good health is 0.9 or less in men and 0.8 or less in women.

The dangers of fat

Each time you eat an extra 3500 calories over and above your body's energy needs, it will lay down 500 g (1 lb) of stored fat. Your body does need some fat to help it regulate its temperature. Fat also cushions and insulates your tissues and organs and serves as your main form of stored energy should you need to call on it. Ideally, though, that fat should only be 8 to 22 per cent of your total body weight if you're a man and 21 to 34 per cent if you're a woman.

If both your BMI rating and your waist circumference suggest that you're overweight, it's not just a matter of needing to lose weight so you can fit into your favourite dress or do your belt up an extra notch. Carrying excess fat puts your body at a considerable risk of serious ill-health. As you gain weight, you are at an increased risk of high blood pressure, coronary heart disease, type II diabetes, osteoarthritis and several forms of cancer. In fact, if you're clinically obese you're twice as likely to die of heart disease. Obese men are 33 per cent more likely to die of a form of cancer and obese women are 50 per cent more likely to develop breast cancer and 27 times more at risk of developing diabetes.

There are also less physically serious but equally distressing conditions, such as bladder-control problems, gallstones, sleep disturbances, infertility, circulatory problems and back pain, which are all pretty likely the more overweight you become.

Factor in the psychological effects of being fat in our society and the picture is even darker. In our world, slim equals not only beautiful, but happy and successful. If you're overweight, you're judged as lazy, less intelligent and lacking in self-control. That lays the ground for some potentially damaging psychological effects should you happen to put on some extra weight. As we'll see, the whole realm of weight and dieting is fraught with a worrying combination of self-loathing and low self-esteem, which can propel us into dangerously disordered attitudes to eating.

What's on offer

Let's take a look at the bewildering array of diets available to someone wanting to lose a few kilos. While for many years most diets were founded on calorie-counting and eating low-fat, high-carbohydrate foods, things have changed. A lot more extreme fad-type diets emerged. How about the cabbage soup diet, which suggests you exist almost entirely on boiled cabbage for days at a time? Or there's the blood group diet, which determines what you should be eating on the basis of your blood type. Other fads included meal-replacement milkshakes, diet pills or even appetite-suppressing supplements.

More recently, the infamous Atkins diet hit the headlines worldwide, representing a growing trend towards low-carbohydrate, high-protein, high-fat diets. Following in Dr Atkins' footsteps was the Zone Diet, which advocates that your food should be 40 per cent carbohydrates, 30 per cent fat and 30 per cent protein. Then there was Sugar Busters, which said 30 per cent carbohydrates, 40 per cent fat and 30 per cent protein ought to do the trick. With this ever-increasing selection of different 'solutions' now available, where on earth

Case Study
The diet addict

Helen is in her late twenties and wants to lose 10 kg (22 lb). 'If you took 365 days of the year, I'm probably on a diet for 320 of them. When I'm on a diet I feel in control but I've tried every diet known and as soon as I come off them, the weight just goes back on.' Being a chronic dieter has seriously affected Helen's feelings about her weight. 'The first thing I do when I wake up is think about whether or not I'm feeling fat that day and if I am then the whole day's affected.' All her friends and family feel that Helen is overly concerned about her weight and that it's affecting her everyday life. Each time she tries and gives up on another diet, she ends up feeling worse about herself and even accepts that her view of her own weight is probably distorted now as a result.

With the support of her friends and her partner, Helen is now working to improve her body image and is gradually learning to accept the way she looks. 'Acknowledging that a large part of the problem is down to my distorted view of my body has helped a lot. Now I'm trying to be more realistic about my ideal weight and I'm not pinning my hopes on faddy diets any more.'

Rate your weight wellbeing

Take our specially designed test to assess how your eating habits and weight are contributing to your overall health:

1 What is your body mass index or BMI? (For details of how to work this out see page 34.)
Under 20 = 0 points
20 to 25 = 1 point
25 to 30 = 2 points
30 or above = 3 points
Your score ☐

2 What is your waist circumference measurement?
Men: less than 86 cm (34 inches) = 1 point
Men: less than 102 cm (40 inches)
= 2 points
Men: 102 cm or more (40 inches or more)
= 3 points
Women: less than 76 cm (30 inches)
= 1 point
Women: less than 88 cm (35 inches)
= 2 points
Women: 88 cm or more (35 inches or more)
= 3 points
Your score ☐

3 How often do you choose low-fat foods over high-fat foods?
Always, I refuse to eat anything but low-fat
= 0 points
Most of the time = 1 point
Sometimes = 2 points
Hardly ever = 3 points
Your score ☐

4 If a plate of food is put in front of you for a meal, how often would you eat all the food on it?
Never = 0 points
It depends on whether I feel full or not
= 1 point
Usually = 2 points
Always = 3 points
Your score ☐

5 If you felt hungry between meals, what would you be most likely to choose as a snack?
I don't snack between meals = 0 points
A handful of nuts or a yoghurt = 1 point
A sandwich, bun or biscuits = 2 points
A chocolate bar = 3 points
Your score ☐

6 How often do you eat processed foods, such as pre-prepared meals or fast food?
Never, I wouldn't consider it = 0 points
Very rarely = 1 point
Once or twice a week = 2 points
Every day = 3 points
Your score ☐

7 How often do you think about your weight?
All the time – if I put on weight I get very upset = 0 points
Regularly – I don't want to be overweight
= 1 point
Occasionally – I need to lose a bit = 2 points
Never – it's best not to think about it
= 3 points
Your score ☐

8 **How often do you exercise (so that you're slightly breathless)?**
More than 150 minutes each week = 0 points
About 90 minutes each week = 1 point
About 30 minutes each week = 2 points
I don't exercise = 3 points

Your score ☐

Add up your scores and enter your total here ☐

What your score means:
1 to 6 = You take your weight very seriously, perhaps a bit too seriously. Try not to be too hard on yourself and remember that food is one of life's great pleasures. You should try to find ways to enjoy it and be a healthy weight without being so strict about your diet and exercise regime. Consult a nutritionist for specific advice on a new eating plan.

7 to 14 = Keep up the good work. You have a healthy attitude towards your weight and are sticking to good eating and exercise habits to maintain it.

15 to 18 = It's likely that your eating habits need a good rethink. Read through our top tips for weight loss (see pages 40–2) and also the top tips for healthy eating in Chapter 1 (see page 14). Specifically try to cut down on high-fat, high-sugar food, such as ready meals and refined carbohydrates. Try to increase the amount of exercise you do each week to around 90 minutes.

19 to 24 = Your diet and eating habits need urgent changes. If you carry on in this vein, there's a good chance you will go on to develop health problems (if you haven't already) as a result of the extra weight you're carrying. Consult a doctor or nutritionist as soon as possible and resolve to change your ways.

do you turn when you want to shift those extra kilos? In thousands of cases, people are so desperate to lose weight that they'll try as many different diets as possible, each time hoping that it is going to be the magic bullet that will help them achieve the weight loss they long for. But before we go any further, let's look at the fundamental flaws that exist in the whole concept of fad diets.

The truth about diets

It's a staggering fact that 95 per cent of all diets fail. When our stone-age bodies were first designed, food supply wasn't exactly reliable. So the human body evolved an emergency mode of holding on to its stored energy when less food was available – and we've inherited that. So your body registers a crash diet as a time of famine and slows down the rate at which the calories you do eat are burned up, making it even harder to lose weight. But it gets worse: your physiology means that going on that diet could eventually make you more overweight – that's because when you give up on the diet, your stone-age body tries to make the most of the plentiful food by piling on more fat than usual as a precaution for the future. This is why so many people get themselves stuck in a cycle of yo-yo dieting.

Aside from our physiology, it's worth considering how dieting can affect your feelings about food – and how they can have knock-on effects on your weight. In an early psychological study from the 1950s, a group of normal-weight men were fed only 75 per cent of their normal food intake so that they lost about a quarter of their body weight. Intriguingly, the researchers noticed that the men became increasingly obsessed with food – they collected recipes, put up posters of food and one even planned to become a

chef. They also reported feeling much more irritable and moody. After the study had ended and their body weight was restored, many of the subjects felt they had lost control of their eating patterns. They would regularly binge on 'desirable' foods when they could and had much greater difficulty keeping to a stable weight.

By imposing strict restrictions on your daily food through a diet plan, it seems you're almost setting yourself up for failure. Canadian researchers have recently studied chronic yo-yo dieters to get to the bottom of this, with fascinating results. In a typical laboratory set-up, the subjects (usually female) are split into two groups and given either a fattening milkshake or no food at all. Then both groups are given three flavours of a different food (such as ice cream, biscuits and nuts) with the instruction to rate these for taste. In fact, the researchers are secretly recording how much food each subject eats while making her taste ratings. What you find is that, out of the group who were given a milkshake, those people who are currently on a diet eat more of the ice cream, biscuits and nuts than the non-dieters. Once that milkshake has broken their diet plan, the dieter feels that they're now free to overindulge. Interestingly, this effect also occurs when dieters drink alcohol or are in a subdued mood.

If you're overweight, the likelihood is that you'll already have negative feelings about yourself and your body – that's what our culture imposes on 'fat people'. In the eyes of our society, overweight people have failed – by eating too much, by not controlling themselves, by not having the willpower to get rid of the weight. So with those sorts of

Right: Making exercise a part of your life will boost your self-esteem and improve your body shape.

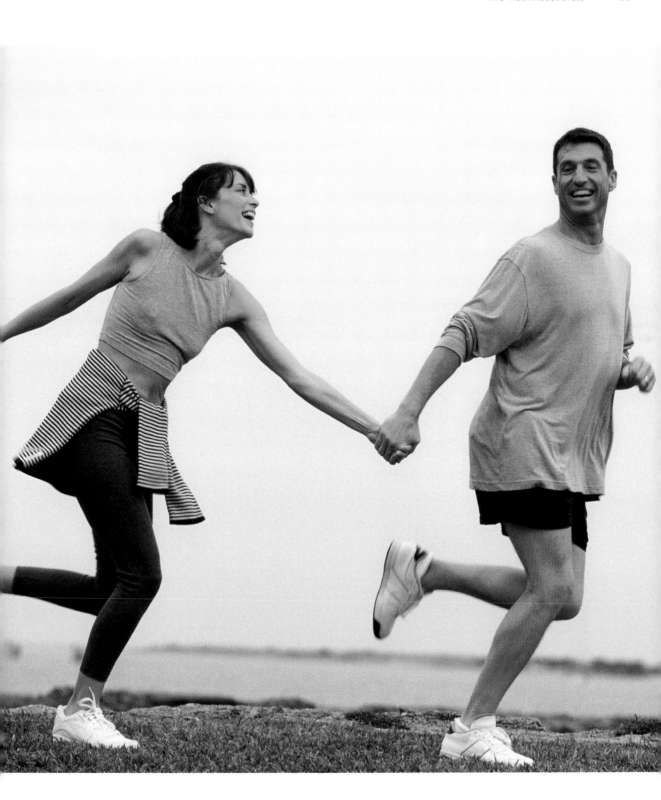

Top tips for losing weight

- **Write a food diary.** Keep an honest record of everything you eat and drink for one week. It might sound simple but studies show that the vast majority of people unconsciously under-report how much they're eating. Once you factor in those French fries you ate off your partner's plate, the biscuits someone was passing round at the office, or the children's leftovers, your daily calorific intake is likely to be a lot more than you imagined. Seeing what you've eaten over a whole week in black and white is also helpful to work out how to balance your diet better.

- **Write an exercise diary.** Think carefully about how much exercise you do over a week – and don't forget to include activities you might not think of as exercise: running for the bus, walking to the train station each day or walking the dog.

- **Be realistic.** Once you know what you're really eating and how much energy your body is actually expending, you need to work out ways to reduce the former and increase the latter. But it has to be a plan that will fit in with your everyday life, otherwise the chances are that you will simply give up on it – and feel worse about yourself. There is no point planning to go to the gym three times a week if you can only spare an hour a week. Likewise, if you are a working mother, what are the chances that you'll have time to prepare special diet meals for yourself every day? Improving your eating and exercise behaviour in small ways every day won't lead to a quick overall weight loss, but see it as taking feasible steps to getting to your goal weight gradually – and staying there.

- **Eat just a little bit less.** If you fall into the overweight category based on your BMI and waist circumference (see page 34), you need to tailor your food intake to 1500 calories a day if you're a man and 1200 calories a day if you're a woman. Aim to lose no more than 1 kg (2 lb) a week – it might not sound like much but if you're losing any more the chances are you're restricting your eating in a way that won't be sustainable over the long term. (If you fall into the obese category, it's best that you see your doctor or a nutritionist to help you lose weight safely.)

- **Fight the desire to lose weight quickly.** Yes, it's true people can lose weight quickly on fad diets, particularly the Atkins diet, where very low-carb, high-fat food is consumed, but remember that crash diets don't offer a sustainable eating plan for the long term. It can be very alluring to see skinny celebrities advocating their low-carb diets as a way of life, but don't be fooled. Hollywood's leading ladies aren't tucking into bacon and eggs every morning for their breakfast. The chances are they're eating a low-carb and low-fat diet, which is simply a (very extreme) reflection of that simple equation – eat less than your body needs to lose weight. Nevertheless, back in the real world, bear in mind that while you're keeping your fat intake low, that doesn't mean you can eat unlimited amounts of carbohydrate to compensate, so most of us probably do need to cut down on the carbs a bit. But remember that any diet that recommends cutting right down on one whole food group and overeating another (as Atkins does with carbs and fats) is going to carry health risks. It is far better for your body to lose weight slowly and sensibly. Use our tips for healthy meals in Chapter 1 (see page 14) for advice on how you can eat a more balanced diet.

● **Why are you hungry?** It's true that we feel the need to eat for many different reasons other than physical hunger, as we saw in Chapter 1. Try to identify the difference between your desire to eat when you really need to and when you're experiencing other emotions that may have become linked to your hunger. It's also worth bearing in mind that sometimes your body can confuse thirst for hunger. If you feel like eating between meal times, try having a glass of water and waiting for a few minutes to see if the hunger feelings subside. Also, remember that some foods will make you feel full for longer – for example small amounts of monounsaturated fats like olive oil. Other foods will trigger your hunger – if you eat sugary food, it will cause a huge surge in your blood sugar. Your body will take emergency action to reduce this, which will cause you to feel hungry – you may well have experienced this after eating carbohydrate- and sugar-rich foods, such as pasta, white bread or sweets. Learn to use food to your advantage and snack on protein-rich foods (such as low-fat cheese or a handful of almonds or hazelnuts), which turn off your body's hunger signals quickly.

● **Think about the size of your meals.** Limiting your food intake doesn't mean you have to exist on a hugely restrictive diet. Try just serving yourself smaller portions of food. Another way to look at it is that you don't always have to finish what's on your plate. The chances are you're eating more than

your body needs just because it's there. That doesn't mean you're greedy, though. In a fascinating study, scientists fed a group of people soup from normal bowls. They measured what each person ate as a normal portion. Then the next day the experiment was repeated but the bowls were replaced with 'trick' bowls that were secretly re-filled from a hidden reservoir under the table, so that the soup never ran out as the subjects ate it. Whether or not the person was slim or overweight, the continual presence of soup in the bowl made them all eat more than their usual portion size. But when the researchers revealed the secret of the trick bowl to the participants, they noted that in the following day's test, the slimmer subjects adjusted their portion size so that it was closer to the amount of soup they had originally consumed before the trick bowl had been used, while the overweight subjects continued to eat a bigger portion than they first had. It seemed that they simply couldn't resist the sight and smell of the extra soup in the trick bowl. Many of us were trained as young children to finish what was put in front of us – that could now be one of the main reasons why we eat too much.

● **Let yourself have treats.** Reward yourself for healthy eating with the occasional food treat. If you have a biscuit or a chocolate bar once in a while, enjoy it and don't let it trigger feelings of failure or weakness, which might lead you into bad eating habits over a long period. You could try eating healthily during weekdays and then letting yourself have a few more treats at the weekend. Always identify what the treat is going to be and don't eat more of it than you first set out to. Accept that on certain occasions, you might eat more calories than you need, for instance at a special dinner or during the Christmas holidays. Learn to be flexible and adapt your eating habits so that you can enjoy some of these food pleasures and then eat a bit less after they're finished to make up for them. Don't let them trigger a descent into bad eating patterns every day. If you plan ahead to enjoy limited treats, you will feel rewarded and stop feelings of failure and worthlessness rising up.

● **Make exercise a regular part of your life.** There's no way round it. Lack of physical activity is probably the greatest reason why obesity figures are rising. You do need to increase your activity levels if you want to lose weight, but it's also good for your all-round health and wellbeing. As most of us have non-physical jobs, it's easy to become disassociated from your body. Getting back in touch with it with exercise will increase your self-esteem and feelings of control as well as your energy levels, metabolism and overall fitness. Don't despair though, you don't have to go to the gym for hours at a time. Just make sure you get your heart rate up – so that you're slightly breathless – for a good 30 minutes at least three times a week. If you can add in strength training at the gym with weights, even better. Don't hide behind lack of time or hatred of gyms as excuses not to exercise at all. You could go on a 30-minute run or cycle ride around your local area, or try swimming or a dance class. Even

a brisk walk will do, but make sure you get your heart rate up. Try increasing the speed at which you do everyday chores, such as running up the stairs or walking to work.

● **Don't get obsessed by the scales.** It's pointless to torture yourself every day on the scales. Your weight can fluctuate by half a kilo here and there due to variation in water levels (and hormonal changes if you're female). Instead, try weighing yourself once a week. Remember, if you've increased the amount of strength-training exercises you do, you will have more muscle tissue in your body and, as muscle weighs more than fat, it might take a bit longer to lose excess weight.

● **Improve your self-esteem.** Focus on one part of your body that you like and be proud of it, whether that means wearing the sort of clothes that reveal it more or just enjoying a new-found tone in that area if you've begun exercising recently. Try not to focus only on the problem areas.

● **Ask for help if you feel out of control.** If you're struggling with food, exercise, your weight or any feelings about your body, don't suffer alone. It can be very easy for people who are concerned about their weight and body image to slip into disordered eating habits without realizing. If friends or relatives have expressed concern about your eating, do consider speaking to your doctor or a nutritionist for advice that's tailored to your individual needs.

negative emotions on board, if you then attempt an extremely restrictive quick-fix diet, you are setting yourself up for trouble. If you find the diet difficult to stick to or live with (which, let's face it, almost all of them are), you're more than likely to take a slip into old eating habits, which will simply confirm your fears that you have no willpower and can't lose the weight even though you desperately want to. As we saw in Chapter 1, our bodies are designed to love the taste of sugary, high-fat foods, and faced with feeling increasingly bad about ourselves, many of us will simply turn to food for comfort – another nail in the coffin for achieving a healthy weight and feeling good about ourselves.

The bottom line is that there simply is no quick-fix solution, no magic bullet for weight loss. These diets exist because the market for them is so enormous – there are hugely lucrative profits to be made. The question you need to ask yourself is: could you really live on that diet for life? While it might be possible to achieve weight loss relatively quickly on a fad diet, the chances are most people will simply end up returning to their old eating habits and the weight loss will vanish. To get to a healthy weight and stay that way you need to adopt a long-term plan. Follow our top tips for healthy weight loss on pages 40–2.

Detox diets

In recent years, an entirely different type of diet has become popular. It's not about losing excess fat, weight or even toning up your body. It's about doing a bit of bodily spring-cleaning by adopting a special plan to purify yourself of any nasty toxins. Our bodies accumulate toxins from many different sources. The worst culprits are alcohol, drugs and cigarettes. But even if you're a clean-living soul, you'll still be picking up toxins from the environment. The air we breathe is full of pollutants, mostly produced as a result of fossil fuels being burned as an energy source. You'll also be exposed to toxins in your food, especially if it's not organic. There'll be an assortment of pesticides, herbicides and all manner of agricultural chemicals – and although organic food is much safer in that respect, it's still liable to pick up toxins from the air all around us.

It's not just the outside world that exposes our bodies to toxins. They come from deep within us too. Toxic chemical waste is produced by every one of the billions of cells in your body. That's just a side effect of their everyday chores keeping you alive. Luckily, your body's evolved a number of tricks to keep a check on toxins and start the clean-up when it's needed. Your liver's the leader of the pack: it clears alcohol, drugs and other chemical waste from your bloodstream, filters out bacteria and viruses and even keeps a store of vitamins to keep your body healthy. Your kidneys also have a key role in detoxing, neutralizing and removing natural waste products from your body. Your colon makes sure undigestible waste gets excreted. Finally, there's a whole network of special lymphatic vessels branching right across your body, alongside the blood capillaries and nerve fibres. As you'll see in the illustration on page 49, the tubes of the lymph system act as drainage pipes. They soak up excess fluid that is naturally present around our body cells – and that fluid also contains some of the toxins that have been drawn out from your body's tissues.

The proponents of detox diets and treatments argue that our modern lifestyle is so hectic and toxin-ridden that our bodies can't cope with the amount of internal

Battle of the sexes: fighting fat

If you're female you probably feel you're bombarded with images of skinny models, actresses and celebrities by the media (in fact, it's estimated that city-dwellers might see up to 600 images of such bodies every day). That's bound to have an effect on how you feel about your own weight, but don't think men are getting off lightly any more. Men's magazines are increasingly concerned with how to get the perfect body. We do need to realize, however, that physiological differences between the sexes mean fighting fat is a very different battle if you're male or female. Here are the top five facts that explain why:

1   Women need more body fat than men. This is because they require greater energy reserves should they become pregnant. If a woman drops below the minimum amount of fat her body needs, her periods will usually stop temporarily, as in the case of athletes or dancers who have very low body fat, or women suffering from the eating disorder anorexia nervosa.

2   The male sex hormone testosterone helps men to build muscle rather than to lay down fat. That means it's easier for a man than a woman to tone up in the gym. Another effect of testosterone is that it makes men more likely to put on excess weight around the waist, which in health terms puts you at much higher risk of heart disease than fat located below the waist. This is one of the main reasons that more men die of heart disease than women.

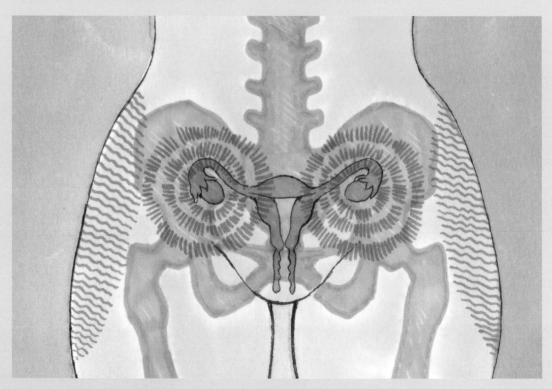

3 For women, the sex hormone oestrogen means that excess fat builds up around the hips and thighs. It's stored there as a nearby source of energy reserves for the body to call upon should a pregnancy occur. Pregnancy usually results in a woman burning up around 80,000 calories over the gestation period to keep herself healthy and her baby developing properly. Interestingly, studies show that pregnant women don't need to 'eat for two' – on average they only need around an extra 300 calories a day. Their bodies compensate for extra energy demands by becoming less active and using energy more efficiently.

4 After the menopause, when a woman's body stops producing the hormone oestrogen, women are more likely to lay fat down around their waist area and so are more at risk of heart disease.

5 Studies show that men tend to lose weight more easily than women because they're less likely to follow a fad diet. They're more likely to sensibly cut back on food portions and increase the amount of exercise they do, while women are more likely to follow a strict restrictive diet, give it up and then begin the whole cycle of dieting again.

Left: At puberty, the ovaries start producing the hormone oestrogen. This triggers the woman's body to store energy reserves on the hips for future pregnancies and also sculpts the typical female hourglass shape.

cleaning there is to do. According to them, the accumulation of both internal and external toxins can lead you to feel tired, sluggish, energyless, and to suffer from digestive problems, allergies, headaches, skin problems – even backaches and swollen joints. So the idea is that you give your body – especially your digestive tract and immune system – a vacation from all the toxins it's struggling to deal with every day. Sounds sensible enough, but let's consider what's involved.

The delights of detoxing

There are a huge number of detox plans to choose from. The simplest (and cheapest) is probably a variety of fasts and restrictive diets. Some advocate that you avoid food altogether for a period of time, surviving only on certain fruit or vegetable juices. Or you could try cutting out certain foods altogether for a while, such as wheat or dairy products. There are also any number of special detox herb powders and drinks that you can incorporate into your daily diet, if you're not so sure about taking on a fast. Whichever you choose, the number one rule tends to be giving up smoking, alcohol and caffeine for a while – an undertaking which can push many people into nasty withdrawal reactions, trigger headaches and make you feel irritable and moody. While detox gurus say that a headache is your first sign that the detox is working – it means toxins are working their way out of your body – there is no scientific evidence to prove that it's not just your body going into a sort of chemical sulk as it pines for its daily morning coffee or the first cigarette of the day.

There are also a number of detox treatments, such as sweating it out in the sauna, which is supposed to drag out even more toxins than usual, or having special

Case Study
The detox diet

Sarah was concerned that her drinking and eating habits were having effects on her body. Filmed by the *Body Hits* team, she embarked on a frugal detox diet plan that involved giving up smoking, alcohol and eating a very limited diet supplemented with special herbs. 'You have to have brown rice every day about three times a day. And after these ten days, I tell you, I'm never going to have brown rice again.' What's more, the herbs didn't go down too well – they had the aroma of 'a pair of stinky socks being boiled'. But the detox did seem to help. 'I started to feel much more healthy and stopped craving chocolate and sweets and I definitely had more energy.' Sarah decided that while the detox plan had been perhaps a bit too extreme, it had taught her that she needed to treat her body with a bit more respect. She now plans to do shorter, more gentle detoxes to give her body a break from time to time.

lymphatic massages to improve your body's own detoxification process. The fluid in your lymph system flows very slowly and unlike your blood supply, it isn't propelled along by your heart. It relies on the movement of your muscles to shift it around. So physically pumping and pushing your lymph fluid around using special massage techniques and products is claimed to help your body clear toxins more efficiently. While these treatments may indeed help, you might want to consider drastically cheaper do-it-yourself options to get your lymph up to speed. We describe these in our top tips for detoxing on pages 48–9.

The most invasive of all the detox therapies is colonic irrigation. It should be performed by a properly trained therapist, who inserts a nozzle into your rectum and then flushes out your colon with a staggering 75–100 litres (16–22 gallons) of purified water mixed with herbs and other cleansing agents. The procedure is supposed to flush out toxic waste matter that has accumulated and is now festering inside your large intestine, creating sluggishness and all-round bad health. Although people do report benefits from the treatment, it's important to note that while it can help chronic constipation (in much the same way as a simple enema), there is no scientific evidence that it does help your body to detoxify. What's more, if you have it done too often or by someone who isn't properly trained, it can be dangerous.

The truth about detox plans
Many people swear by the beneficial effects of detox plans. It's worth bearing in mind that there is currently no scientific evidence to show that they do have physical detoxing effects on your body. However, just because there isn't any hard evidence, that doesn't

mean they don't work at all, although the chances are that people get most of the benefit from the psychological effects of adopting a detox plan. The sense of taking direct control of your body and making a concerted effort to look after it is bound to do some good, just as taking time out from a hectic lifestyle to adjust some of your more unhealthy habits clearly will too. Wellbeing is very much about making time for yourself and your body and finding out whatever it takes to keep yourself healthy in body and soul. If signing up for the occasional frugal fast or diet takes your fancy, then why not? (Although you should always seek medical

Below: The build-up of toxins and waste matter in your gut can cause bacteria to breed, triggering bowel problems and bad health. Some people claim that flushing out the colon with water can help.

Case Study
A bit of colon-cleaning

Giles felt he'd been indulging in too much rich food and wine. A juice fast over several days made him feel better but did result in severe constipation. 'People say you wake up feeling fantastic after a detox, with much more energy – I haven't experienced that yet.' To try and boost the effects, he opted for colonic irrigation. 'I was quite curious about how I'd feel afterwards, but I was more concerned about how uncomfortable it might be!' His fears were put to rest by an experienced therapist and he emerged triumphant. 'I feel fantastic, I really do!' The effects were so positive that he decided he would return for a course of further treatments whenever he was feeling run-down.

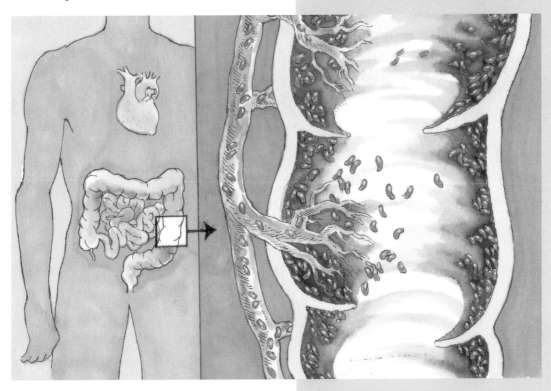

Top tips for detoxing

- **Drink more water.** Your body is constantly losing water – up to 3 litres (5 pints) a day. You breathe out a glass and a bit every day just as water vapour, you sweat out around 750 ml (1¼ pints) even if you're not exercising and you pass over 1.5 litres (2½ pints) in your urine. It's true that you do take in quite a bit from food, but you still need to drink around 1.5 litres (2½ pints, or about eight tall glasses) of water every day just to keep your cells functioning properly. Remember that alcohol and caffeine are diuretics (they make you lose water), so if your day includes either or both, you need to increase your water intake even more. If you make a concerted effort to drink more water, you'll probably notice you have to urinate a bit more frequently at first, but your kidneys will adjust so you won't have to keep running off to the bathroom. Keeping your body hydrated is the number one way to fight toxins and keep everything inside you working smoothly.

- **Cut back on alcohol, cigarettes and caffeine.** If you've made a positive choice to be a drinker, smoker or coffee-drinker, it might not be realistic to suggest giving up these three for the sake of a detoxified body. However, at times when you are feeling run-down or are in ill-health, consider cutting right back on them all for a limited period or if you're feeling particularly strong, cut them out of your life altogether for a while and see if you feel any better. The chances are you'll notice a big improvement that might be a good kickstart to trying to break the habit. And don't forget that carbonated soft drinks, tea and even some herbal teas all contain caffeine too.

- **Be active.** Exercising more will have all-round health benefits as we saw earlier in the chapter. In addition, the more active you are, the more your blood circulation and lymph system will get moving and expel those toxins.

- **Boost your lymph system.** It's true that lymphatic massage can help to stimulate your lymph system to remove toxins that have accumulated in your tissues. But it doesn't have to be an expensive process. Buy a natural-bristle body brush or a loofah from any pharmacy and start dry-brushing your body before every shower or bath. Make sure you always brush in the direction of your heart (so for your lower body that means upwards towards the heart and for your upper body downwards towards it). It's not an unpleasant sensation but it will make your skin a bit red. Don't worry, this is normal. You should notice an improvement in skin smoothness and texture in just a few days too.

- **Catch up on your sleep.** As we'll see in Chapter 4, lack of sleep affects your immune system and challenges all sorts of everyday bodily functions. If things have been a bit hectic lately or you've been sleeping at erratic times, a couple of early nights and slow starts in the morning will boost your energy levels much more than a detox treatment or diet plan. If your schedule doesn't permit catching up on your sleep at night, try and factor in a few 20-minute naps during the day if you can.

- **Wash your fruit and vegetables.** Even if you buy organic produce, always give fruit, vegetables and salad a thorough wash in cold water before you eat them. It won't eliminate all the toxins, but it's a good start.

● **Give your body a treat.** Forget most of the things you might immediately reach for as a treat, such as a chocolate bar or a glass of wine. Think of treating your body for a change – take a long warm candlelit bath or buy yourself a luxurious body cream to keep skin soft and supple. If the benefits of detox treatments are mostly psychological, you can easily recreate them at home by simply finding time to look after your body. A bit of pampering goes a long way.

advice if you are considering undertaking any type of fast, and do make sure it's only a short-term treatment.) Likewise, if you've got the time and money to treat yourself to a detox massage or lymph treatment, you should go ahead and enjoy every minute of it. However, don't be fooled that you can't achieve the same purifying effects yourself by adopting some simple and cheap lifestyle changes. Follow our top tips for detoxing (see opposite) to find out how keeping your body clean and serene doesn't have to mean an expensive treatment or an extreme diet plan.

Below: Your lymph system is a complex network that protects you against infection and keeps the fluid in your body filtered and flowing well. Glands and nodes in your neck, groin and armpits are key parts of the system.

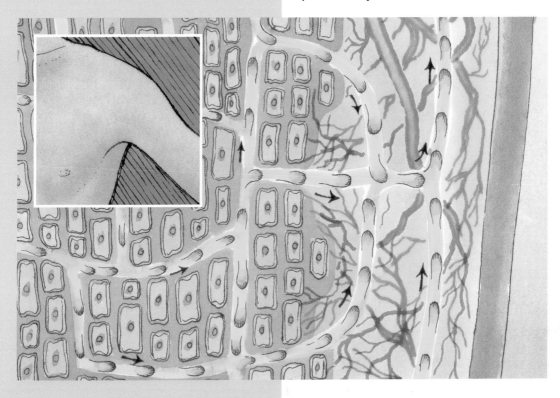

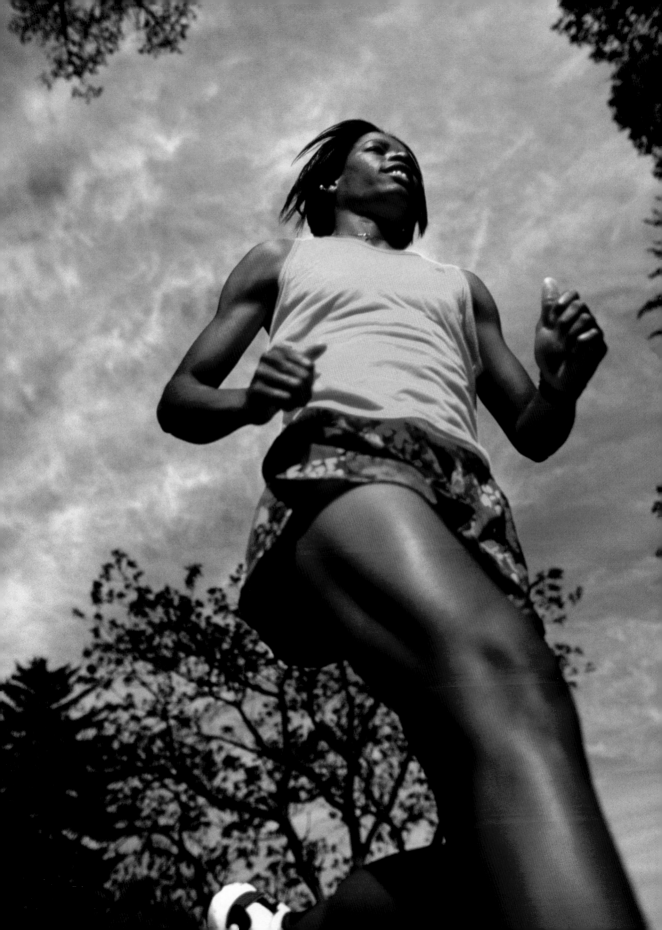

3

Highs & Lows

Imagine a list of the best suggestions for improving health and wellbeing. It would probably read along the lines of: drink less alcohol; give up smoking; stop taking drugs; eat healthier food. Sounds straightforward enough but during the course of today, an astonishing 13 billion alcoholic drinks will be consumed around the world, and in 2003 in the UK alone, more than 3 million people spent a staggering £6.6 billion on illegal drugs. A vast proportion of us seem to be choosing lifestyle habits that are potentially damaging to our physical and mental health. The fact is that some of life's greatest highs carry health risks, but that hasn't stopped human beings everywhere continuously seeking out pleasure and enjoying risk-taking.

In this chapter, we'll look at how we get our kicks from such risky habits as drug-taking. The urge to tinker with our minds has existed for thousands of years, across many different cultures. But it's not only pills and powders that drive our highs – we'll look at natural kicks gained through seemingly positive activities, such as exercise. Whether your poison's illegal or healthy, you need to be aware of what it does (and could potentially do in the long term) to your body and mind to avoid serious health problems.

While our brains have evolved an intricate pleasure system that enables us to enjoy our highs, millions of people around the world also experience the other end of the pleasure spectrum. Lows range from daily stress through panic and anxiety to debilitating depression. We'll reveal what's going on inside the body and brain during these experiences, uncover some of the possible causes and give advice and practical tools to those affected on how to start steering your life back to a happy medium.

Chemical highs

As we saw in Chapter 1, alcohol is the most common and widely used drug of our times. It's also considered far more socially acceptable than the other sorts of mood-altering substances that are available. These other drugs can be grouped into different categories according to their effects. Let's take a look at the most commonly used ones: first, there are substances like cocaine and ecstasy, known as stimulants. Secondly, there are analgesic (pain-killing) drugs, of which heroin is the most notorious and the most harmful. Finally, there's cannabis, which occupies a group of its own and is a relaxant and mild sedative with hallucinogenic potential.

It's estimated that about one in ten people in the UK has taken an illicit drug. Having said that, we don't know the exact levels of drug use with any precision. The latest research suggests each year among 16 to 24 year-olds alone, there are up to 1.6 million users of cannabis; 440,000 users of ecstasy; 275,000 users of cocaine; and at least 34,000 users of heroin.

No-one can have failed to notice that there is huge concern about the use of drugs in our society, and various degrees of legal control exist to alert people to their dangers and to limit their availability and use. You'd think we'd have got the message loud and clear by now that drugs are bad for us: there are all sorts of very obvious downsides related to drug-taking – from ruined lives to family problems to soaring crime rates. Education programmes warn school-age youngsters of the dangers and stories of celebrity drug addictions fill the newspapers on an almost daily basis. Yet thousands upon thousands of people still actively choose to take drugs every day.

The good news is that the vast majority of those who experiment with drugs don't go on to become dependent on them. While the peak period for initiating drug use is between 16 and 20, drug use declines substantially as people get older and large-scale surveys in the US have shown that very few people initiate into use of any illegal drug after they reach 30. That said, the recreational use of drugs is on the increase and in certain social groups it's as socially acceptable as alcohol. But just because you're taking a substance as part of a social activity, that doesn't mean it's harmless or isn't potentially going to have significant long-term effects on your mind and body. If you do take drugs, it's well worth knowing the facts about how they work, so that you can make a more informed choice in the future.

Why take drugs?

Parents are often anxious and exasperated about why their children decide to take drugs. There is a simple reason. Drugs are very effective at changing your mood and making you feel good, or at least different. And for very deep and ancient reasons, human beings do like to alter their mood. Most drugs have some similar effects to alcohol and each one has various specific effects all of their own. But, unsurprisingly, the overall effects of drugs come down to what they do to your brain. And that centres on a neurological feature that is at the very core of how your brain functions in the first place.

Think very small for a second and have a look at the illustration on page 55, which gives you a vastly magnified view of something which is going on inside your head at this very moment. The human brain is the most complex object in the known universe and, as such, its mysterious

Are you dependent on drugs?

Let's look at how doctors assess the extent to which someone has a substance-related problem and whether or not they're dependent. Below are some examples of the sorts of questions asked. Bear in mind that these questions are just the starting point for a thorough assessment that would look more intensively at each individual's situation.

Answer these questions based on your drug-taking over the past 12 months. They apply to any substance. In this example, we'll use cocaine.

1 Have you needed to use more cocaine to get the desired effect or has the same amount had less of an effect?
YES/NO

2 Have you felt sick or unwell when the effects of cocaine wore off or have you taken more of it or a similar drug to relieve or avoid feeling unwell?
YES/NO

3 Have you used cocaine in larger amounts or for a longer period of time than you intended?
YES/NO

4 Have you had a persistent or strong desire to take cocaine?
YES/NO

5 Have you spent a large amount of time obtaining, using or recovering from the effects of cocaine?
YES/NO

6 Have you reduced or given up work, recreational or social activities as a result of your cocaine use?
YES/NO

7 Have you continued to use cocaine despite having physical or psychological problems with it?
YES/NO

If you answered yes to three or more of these questions it's likely you're dependent on the substance. If so, consult a doctor as soon as you can. There are plenty of freely available expert sources of advice and counselling to help and support you on the road to recovery from this dependency (see page 168).

These questions are adapted from the *American Psychiatric Association: Diagnostic and Statistical Manual of Mental Disorders*, Fourth Edition. Washington DC, American Psychiatric Association, 1994.

The facts about drugs

Cannabis

Cannabis comes in many forms and is extracted from the plant *Cannabis sativa*. Most people smoke the drug mixed with tobacco in a joint. There are increasingly strong leaf forms in the UK today. The physical effects include sedation, sleepiness, dilated pupils and increased appetite. The psychological effects include feeling more relaxed, talkative and giggly, although some people become quite introspective and quiet. Long-term use may lead to the user feeling more anxious, depressed and possibly paranoid. If a cannabis-user mixes tobacco in their joints, they're at a similar risk as a normal cigarette smoker of respiratory problems, as well as lung, mouth and throat cancers. Some studies have suggested that the risk may be even higher because joints are smoked without a filter.

Ecstasy

Ecstasy (MDMA) is a synthetically produced stimulant, usually taken recreationally in pill form. It alters levels of serotonin, which is a neurotransmitter in your brain that works in a very similar way to the pleasure chemical dopamine. Serotonin's usual role in the brain includes regulating mood, aggression and sexual activity. Ecstasy (or E) triggers abnormally high levels of serotonin in the synapses of the brain, enabling users to experience an overwhelming feeling of love and happiness, increased confidence and the urge to be in physical contact with people around them. However, increases in heart rate and blood pressure and imbalanced water levels can cause physical problems, and long-term use appears to increase anxiety, depression and paranoia. There is some evidence to suggest it may permanently damage the brain's serotonin system.

Cocaine

Cocaine (benzoylmethylecgonine) is a stimulant that is extracted from the leaves of the plant *Erythroxlon coca*. In the UK, two illegal cocaine products are available: cocaine hydrochloride (a white crystalline salt that comes in powder form) and a whitish crystalline alkaloid form known as crack. The physical effects include increased heart rate, blood pressure and body temperature; the drug also has local anaesthetic properties. The psychological effects of cocaine include elevated mood, increased alertness and the suppression of appetite. Higher doses cause restlessness and very large amounts may lead to erratic and violent outbursts. Long-term dependent users often develop a form of social phobia and become withdrawn and even paranoid. It is unclear whether people experience withdrawal effects when stopping after prolonged use; those who do get symptoms usually complain of fatigue, agitation, depression, anxiety, sleep disturbance and unpleasant dreams. These symptoms usually fade away after a week or so.

Heroin

Heroin is a member of a class of substances called opiates. These include both natural products (e.g. morphine) derived from the poppy (*Papaver somniferum*), semi-synthetic substances (e.g. diamorphine) and synthetic products (e.g. methadone, dihydrocodeine). Heroin, which is a powerful, relatively short-acting analgesic, is the opiate most commonly used by addicts. The physical effects include reduced sensitivity to pain, constricted pupils and drowsiness. The psychological effects include initial euphoria, increased wellbeing and diminished anxiety. At higher doses, users have slurred speech and attention difficulties. A heroin addict who suddenly stops taking the drug will experience severe withdrawal symptoms: distress and anxiety, nausea and vomiting, diarrhoea, muscle aches, fatigue and insomnia. These symptoms usually begin about six hours after the last dose, reach peak intensity between two and three days later and then diminish over the following week.

Below: Between each of your brain cells is a miniscule gap or synapse that nerve messages must get across to work. Chemicals like dopamine, shown here as bright green spheres, ferry the messages from one cell to the next.

workings are unimaginably complicated to most of us. However, what you need to know to understand how drugs work is that your 100 billion brain cells (or neurons) aren't actually physically connected. In between each lies a tiny gap or synapse. For the myriad of messages to get around your brain as they need to do to keep you talking, walking, thinking and creating, your brain chemicals must get across the gaps. Dopamine is the name of one of your key neurotransmitters (chemicals that do cross the gap). Tiny bubbles of dopamine are released from the end of the first cell into the synapse and then get sucked up by special receptors on the receiving cell. The process continues around your brain allowing the messages to be transmitted at lightning speed.

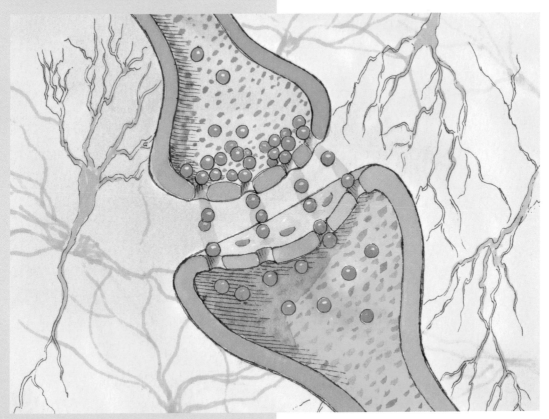

Rewarding highs

The reason why dopamine is a key player in our quest for highs is that the human brain has developed a chemical reinforcement system that rewards us for doing things that are needed for our survival. It was essential that our ancestors didn't grow tired of eating or having sex so a chemical reward got attached to those two vital activities. What that means for you is that when you eat a meal or have sex, your brain rewards you by producing feelings of pleasure, so encouraging you to do this again in the future. Dopamine is the brain's own natural stimulant.

The action of this internal reward system is the reason why all drugs work. If there was no reward system, drugs would have no effect on us at all. So, they hijack the brain's natural pleasure system causing levels of dopamine to build up, stimulating pleasure signals over and over again. And what's more, there are specific areas of the brain called receptors that get fired up when a person takes a particular drug. You're born with these special chemical docking-bays inside your brain – if you take a drug, the substance will head straight to them and fit into them like a key into a lock. Heroin, cocaine, nicotine and alcohol all have these special receptors lying in wait. Once fired up, these trigger dopamine release (as well as other more complex actions that we won't go into). Cannabis is unusual in that it works in the brain via its own unique neurotransmitter called anandamide, but the same principle applies.

The nasty sting in the tail is that over time the brain adapts to being drenched in unnatural dopamine levels and resets itself to produce less and less, forcing the user to increase their drug-dosing to get the same effect. Eventually the system gets so worn

Right: If recreational drugs are part of your lifestyle, it's vital you understand their effects on your body.

down that there's little pleasure to be had at all – it becomes all about the ritual of taking the drug. If someone becomes addicted to certain kinds of drugs – particularly heroin – the body will experience withdrawal symptoms if it doesn't receive regular doses. The vicious circle that can trap people and turn them into addicts starts with the desire for pleasure which, when gratified by drugs, leads to ever-diminishing production of natural pleasure chemicals in the brain, resulting in the physiological need to top up the body with regular doses of a drug.

Assess your drug use

If you use drugs, it's worth assessing how they might be affecting you. Turn back to Chapter 1 and the questionnaire entitled 'Rate your relationship with alcohol' on page 28. Complete it again, but this time substitute the drug you use for the word alcohol in each question. If you use more than one drug, complete the questionnaire separately for each one.

What your score means:

0 to 3 = You are using the drug at a very low level but it's still definitely worth thinking about the health risks you're taking – not to mention the financial costs.

4 to 26 = You should definitely try to stop or in the first instance, at least cut down. Most people who need to do something about their drug use find that stopping altogether is the best approach; but if you feel this is not for you, then work through our strategy for controlling alcohol use on pages 30–1 and apply it to your drug-taking.

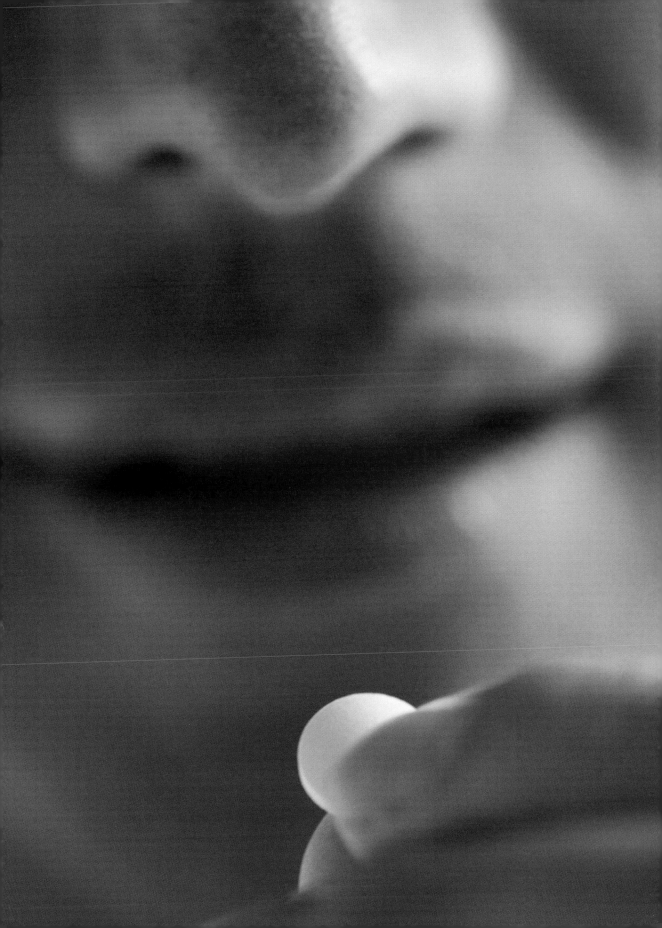

27 or more = You need to see a doctor or a specialist treatment agency for advice tailored just for you. Turn to page 168 for details of confidential telephone lines or organizations you could contact.

A natural buzz

Delving into drugs isn't the only way to get high. Scientists have shown that when you exercise, the pituitary gland in your brain (see the illustration below) releases morphine-like chemicals called endorphins. It's believed that these are pumped out of the brain and into

Below: When you exercise, the pituitary gland in your brain (seen here in pink) pumps out endorphins, your body's own morphine-like painkillers. Many scientists believe these are responsible for the mood boost you get from exercise.

your central nervous system (CNS) and bloodstream to help relieve any pain brought about by exercising. For decades, a debate has raged over whether they're also responsible for bringing about feelings of euphoria or wellbeing after exercising known as 'the runner's high'. It's very difficult to measure levels of endorphins in the CNS and the jury's still out on whether or not the feel-good effects of exercise are down to these mysterious chemicals.

Another possibility is that the mood-lifting properties of working out are not so much down to physiological reactions but more about an all-round psychological boost. When you exercise, you're having time out from your daily life and all the concerns and worries that come with it. You're also taking part in an activity that is widely regarded as

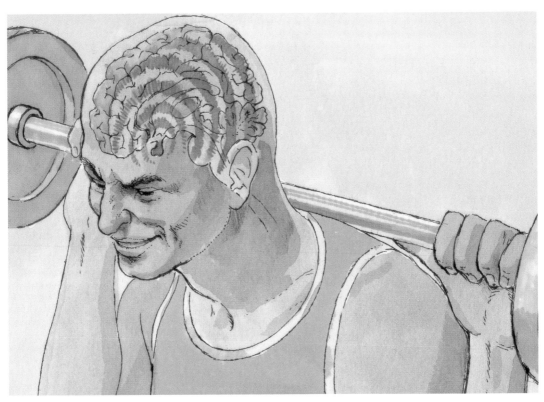

positive and beneficial for your health, so it is bound to do your self-esteem and sense of self-control the power of good. In addition, as we saw in Chapter 2, taking regular exercise is a highly effective way of improving your physical health too: it boosts your metabolism and circulation, reduces weight gain and keeps your body – in particular, your heart – healthy. The chances are that the exercise high is an intricate mix of the chemicals being released inside you combined with positive feelings of reward and wellbeing. With time,

that creates a positive state of mind that is reinforced each time you exercise again.

It just goes to show that you can achieve physical and mental highs without resorting to taking substances like alcohol or drugs, which carry all those undesirable health risks. But don't be fooled, any high has dangers attached and that applies to the natural kick of exercise too. You can get addicted to working out and, as many people are now discovering, that can have devastating effects on your mind, body and lifestyle.

Top tips for keeping exercise under control

- **Acknowledge the problem.** If exercise is controlling your life, the chances are you're already sick of friends and family members nagging you about overdoing it – and time after time, you've probably denied they're right. Don't feel ashamed to admit things have got out of control. Admitting it is the first step to getting over it.

- **Get help.** Ask your doctor to refer you to a psychologist or counsellor who can help you get better. Don't struggle on alone.

- **You'll still be able to work out.** Once you've decided you want to take steps to deal with the addiction, your counsellor or therapist might suggest that you give up exercise completely for a period of around four weeks. That probably fills you with horror right now, but during that time, you'll do some intensive work on the problem that will help redefine how you think about exercise. Gradually, you should be able to start re-introducing exercise into your lifestyle – albeit in much smaller doses.

- **Think about fitness, not appearance.** Try to concentrate on some realistic fitness goals, rather than focusing on the 'more is better' concept. Start trying to see exercise as being more about your fitness and overall health than what it's doing to your physical appearance.

- **Take advice from a personal trainer.** Work out a programme together that's both safe and effective. Ask the trainer or other gym staff to keep an eye on you over the coming months, so you don't slip back into bad habits.

- **Treat your body with respect.** Your body has evolved to feel pain so that it protects you from being exposed to any further damage or harm. Under no circumstances should you exercise when you've got an injury or are unwell. Start listening to your body and try to understand its limits when it comes to physical exertion. Likewise, start factoring in rest days between exercising sessions to give your body time to recover.

Case Study
The thrill of exercise

Phil, 31, openly acknowledges that exercise has become something of a problem for him. 'When I was much younger, I put on a lot of weight and got teased for it. I tried every diet under the sun and eventually resorted to secretly making myself sick to keep my weight under control.' Phil knew he had to do something about his bulimia and started working out at the gym instead. He felt better about his body and more in control, but his new-found passion for exercise got out of hand. He now goes to the gym every day without fail, monitors his weight and each work-out obsessively and puts exercise ahead of everything else in his life. 'I'd say it was the cause of my marriage break-up: I could have been working on our problems, but I was always down at the gym instead.' If he can't get to the gym, the panic sets in. 'I get sweaty palms, start to feel fat and on occasions I've even resorted to my bulimia again as a way of feeling in control.' Phil is in a new relationship now and is trying to tackle his addiction day by day with help from a support group.

Addicted to exercise

It's not known how many people suffer from this addiction, but as increasing numbers of people take up exercise to improve their overall health, so more are falling prey to a compulsion to exercise. So what defines a normal healthy attitude to working out and what symptoms reflect a passion gone too far? Take our simple test to find out if your exercise style means trouble.

Circle true or false for each of the following statements.

1 I try to work out every day if at all possible. TRUE/FALSE
2 If I absolutely have to miss a workout, I will do double the amount the following day or whenever I can. TRUE/FALSE
3 If I'm ill or have an injury, I'll still do everything in my power to get my workout done that day. TRUE/FALSE
4 If I can't exercise for whatever reason, I tend to feel anxious, guilty, irritable or upset. TRUE/FALSE
5 Friends or family have suggested that I don't need to exercise so much. TRUE/FALSE
6 In the past I have cancelled social arrangements or missed work so that I can exercise. TRUE/FALSE

If you've answered true to any of the statements, you should re-assess your exercise habits. The more statements you've agreed with, the more you need to make that re-assessment a priority. Overdoing it carries a number of serious health risks, ranging from painful injuries, such as torn muscles, tendons and ligaments, right through to permanently weakened joints or even stress fractures in bones. What's more, if your body as a whole is under excessive exercise stress, your immune system is likely to become suppressed, leaving you at risk of serious infections. When exercise addiction gets out of control, it can literally take over your mind and your life, as the case study opposite shows. Bear in mind that experts often consider an addiction to exercise as being very similar to eating disorders, such as anorexia and bulimia. If you're suffering from an addiction to exercise, there's every chance that your body image and self-esteem will be very low. You may have even developed symptoms of eating disorders as well. Read our top tips for overcoming exercise addictions on page 59, but don't rely on them alone – your recovery will be helped enormously by you seeking medical or psychological help. Turn to page 168 for further information on how to find a therapist or counsellor in your local area.

Everyday lows

While more of us complain about being 'stressed' each day, what does the term actually mean to our bodies? While we might think of stress as part and parcel of modern life with all its everyday pressures, the human body has evolved an intricate response to stressful situations over thousands of years. Let's uncover what really goes on inside your body when you encounter stress.

Imagine you're on your way home, walking down a dark street at the end of an evening out. It's quiet, apart from one shady-looking figure up ahead of you. You're probably

Below: Above each of your kidneys sits an adrenal gland (shown here in yellow). In a stressful situation, these produce the chemicals adrenaline and cortisol as part of the human 'fight or flight' reaction.

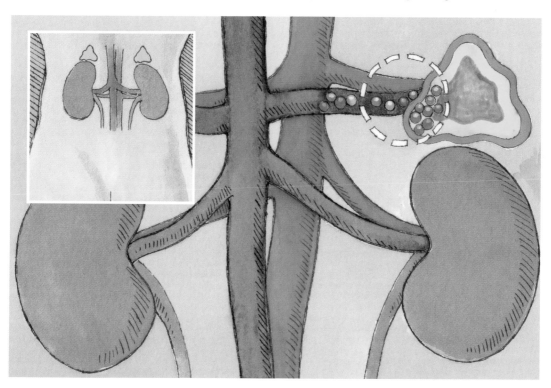

feeling a little cautious – concerned, even – and eager to get home as soon as possible. Meanwhile, inside your brain and body, a veritable cacophony of chemical messages and reactions is going on. First, the potentially dangerous situation you've found yourself in will have triggered the sensory areas of your brain's cortex to send emergency messages to a tiny almond-shaped bit of your brain called the amygdala. It's responsible for sensing threats and fearful situations. It will have started a high-speed chemical relay race inside your body, nudging your hypothalamus to release what's known as corticotopin-releasing hormone (CRH). In turn, that triggers your pituitary gland to pump out another chemical, adrenocorticotropin (ACTH). Finally, this mind-bogglingly complex chemical domino-effect reaches your adrenal glands, which sit just above your kidneys. These glands are the seat of your body's main stress response. As you'll see in the illustration on page 61, they produce two key hormones: adrenaline and cortisol, which pour out into your bloodstream. Adrenaline boosts your reaction time and increases your blood pressure and heart rate, diverting your blood to your muscles. Cortisol releases glucose (sugar) and fatty acids from your body's emergency reserves to power your muscles and brain. Your breathing becomes fast and shallow, your senses are sharpened, you are alert and you can feel your heart racing in your chest. This is the core of the body's 'fight or flight' response – in other words, the chemical reaction enables you to flee or confront the source of danger in a life-threatening situation.

As it happens, the shady figure up ahead of you turns out to be a harmless old man taking his dog out for an evening walk. You sail past and carry on, reaching your home safe and sound. As the perceived threat passes, your body's cortisol levels reach a peak and trigger a protective feedback system inside your brain. It dampens down the release of adrenaline and cortisol, bringing your hormone levels back down to normal again.

Put like that, the body's stress response sounds like a cleverly effective system – and in the time of our ancient ancestors, it certainly was. They lived in an extremely dangerous environment with little protection, stability or security. The 'fight or flight' response evolved as a way of boosting survival chances in the occasional life-or-death situation. But therein lies our main problem with stress: while the dark, dangerous street example could potentially have been a life-threatening situation, the vast majority of stressful episodes we encounter in everyday life tend to be mental, emotional or abstract – and those occur far more than just occasionally. You might worry about whether you'll be able to pay the rent; be concerned about why you and your partner are arguing so much; or even stress about whether or not nuclear war will break out in the future. The fact is that whether you're facing a potential attacker or fretting about financial, emotional and family issues, your body is undergoing precisely the same life or death stress response – and over time, that can wreak havoc on the health of your mind and body.

Effects of stress

During your body's stress response, the surge in your blood pressure – designed to drive you out of a dangerous situation – increases the amount of force exerted on your arteries. The extra supplies of glucose and fatty acids

Top tips for beating stress

• **Make time for yourself.** Try to set aside 30 minutes a day for relaxation or simply thinking time. Even if you do nothing during that time, it doesn't matter – it's very important that you have time to rest from your hectic daily schedule.

• **Learn to say no.** Our culture puts an enormous pressure on us to enjoy our careers, social lives, homes and families, and it can be difficult to juggle all these elements. If you're the kind of person whose diary is always full and maybe even double-booked, you need to find ways of making more time for yourself. That will probably mean saying no to some of your social arrangements or the less important work commitments.

• **Set realistic goals.** We often create a lot of stress for ourselves by expecting too much. If you have a list of things you need to do, be realistic about how many you can comfortably get done in a day or how much work you'll need to put in to meet a deadline without a mad panic. Likewise, allow yourself enough time to get to appointments, meetings and arrangements. There's nothing like time ticking away to fire up your stress response.

• **Don't put your body under more stress.** When times are tough, we're far more likely to turn to bad habits and start overdoing alcohol, smoking or even drug-taking. You might binge on unhealthy foods or indulge in caffeine. While all these seem to relieve tension at the time, ultimately they are simply putting your body under more stress and are all likely to compromise your sleep, a vital weapon in combating stress.

• **Get enough sleep.** As we'll see in Chapter 4, stress and sleep are intricately linked through the action of the hormone cortisol. You may find it hard to sleep if you're stressed as high cortisol makes it difficult for us to feel sleepy, but don't get caught in a stress-insomnia trap. Follow our sleep tips on page 78 to make sure you get ample rest for your body and mind.

• **Breathe deep.** You need to find a way to relax that suits you best and try to incorporate it into your 30 minutes of time set aside for yourself each day. If you're interested in meditation, give it a go. Otherwise, simply try taking a very deep breath in, holding it for four seconds then blowing it out very gradually. Try deep breathing for a good few minutes or find ways to relax your body through stretching or gradually letting tension fall away from each of your muscles and joints.

• **Exercise.** It has been shown as one of the best ways to burn off stress chemicals and all that extra energy produced by the body's stress response. It also produces a feel-good effect, as we saw earlier, and improves mood and self-esteem (as well as overall health and fitness). Be careful not to overdo it though – exercising too much triggers the body to produce even more cortisol. Moderation is the key.

• **Ask for help.** If you've tried all the tips above and still feel that stress is affecting your mental and physical health, it's time to take further action. Consider speaking to a therapist or counsellor – even one or two sessions could help you find new ways of coping.

mobilized by the stress hormone cortisol to increase your energy eventually get to excess levels in your bloodstream. If you're not in a strictly life-or-death situation, but just worrying about something, all that extra energy doesn't get used up and is left to accumulate inside you. Over time, that takes the form of fatty deposits inside your arteries, which narrow your blood vessels and gradually starve your heart of oxygen, putting you at risk of heart disease, heart attacks and strokes. There are also thought to be links between high levels of stress and many forms of cancer, but these aren't yet fully understood.

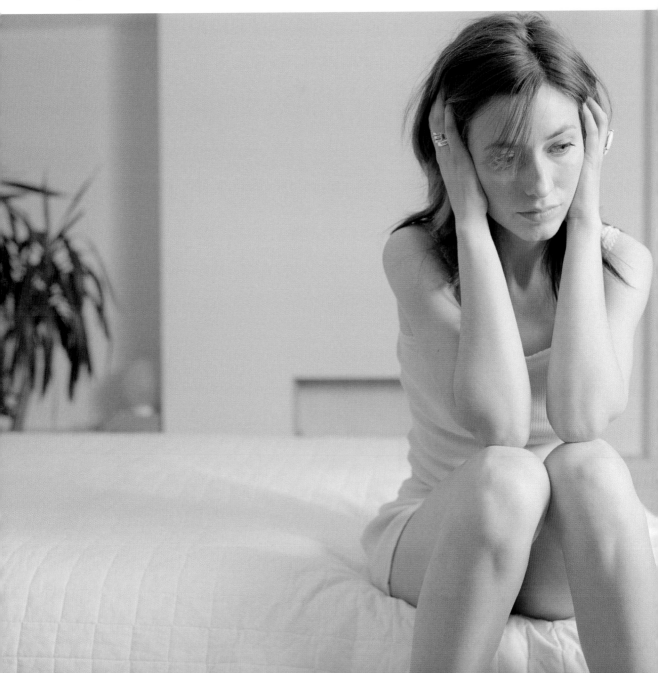

If the stress reaction becomes routine inside the body, increased cortisol levels also suppress your immune system and affect your blood sugar levels and metabolism leading to weight gain. Cortisol has also been shown to kill off brain cells in your hippocampus – a small seahorse-shaped structure in your brain that stores and processes memories – and as we'll see later on in this chapter, it can even trigger anxiety and depression.

But perhaps most worryingly of all, new scientific research has shown that stress can actually rewire your brain and alter its chemical response. In other words, you can become sensitized to stress, so that with time, your body won't respond to it in the same way in the future. You could become so super-sensitive to stressful situations through repeated exposure to them in the past or through one particularly traumatic event that your body unleashes the ferocious 'fight or flight' response inappropriately when things aren't that bad at all – with all sorts of damaging effects on your body. In a fascinating study, American researchers interviewed two groups of veterans of the Second World War and found that among those who had been taken as prisoners of war, the number who had gone on to have a stroke over 50 years later was eight times higher than among those who hadn't been captured. It was as if the first group's brains had been rewired after their severe trauma and had gone on to respond to stress excessively ever since, resulting in their eventual strokes. The study concluded that stress was a far greater risk factor for stroke than almost anything else, even high blood pressure.

Left: If you feel stressed or anxious, it's well worth asking your doctor about medication or therapy.

It's believed that stressful events that occur at a young age have particular power to sensitize a person to stress. If you had a very unstable home environment when you were growing up or one of your parents died when you were a young age, the chances are that your stress reaction will have been affected by that. Some of us might also be genetically predisposed to responding to stressful situations more strongly than others. Whatever your own personal stress reaction, it's vital for your health and wellbeing that you try to minimize the effects of stress on your mind and body. Use our top tips on page 63, which are designed not only to help you avoid stress but also to deal with it better when it does hit you.

When worry takes over

While mild pressure and tension are accepted parts of most of our lifestyles, chronic stress is clearly a problem. In much the same way, the occasional feelings of worry – say, if you have to give a speech or go on a date – are also part of normal everyday human experience. But when worry gets out of hand, you could be in for trouble. Most people don't realize it, but anxiety is a recognized psychological disorder – and millions of people all over the world suffer from it. The link between stress and anxiety is a strong one; if your stress response gets sufficiently sensitized by a traumatic event or ongoing chronic stress, you could be tipped into an anxiety disorder that causes severe distress and disrupts your life. We're talking about situations in which anxiety becomes a constant and controlling force in people's lives. In the grip of anxiety, it's often hard to separate the sort of behaviour that you might think of as 'normal' from feelings that you should consider getting medical help and treatment for. If you're concerned that anxiety may be affecting your life either mildly or significantly, answer our checklist of anxiety disorder symptoms below:

1 Do you have regular worries and fears in one or more areas, such as health or money? YES/NO

2 Do you ever have a strong feeling that something bad is about to happen? YES/NO

3 Do your worries ever interfere with your daily routines, for example sleeping or eating, or make it hard for you to concentrate? YES/NO

4 Do you feel you get unnecessarily worried about everyday activities, but can't stop yourself? YES/NO

5 Do you find yourself carrying out endless checks and rechecks of simple actions you've already completed, such as turning lights off or locking doors? YES/NO

6 Do you ever experience feelings of fear or worry for no particular reason? YES/NO

7 Have you ever experienced sudden feelings of panic, breathlessness, dizziness and terror for no apparent reason? YES/NO

If you answered yes to questions 1, 2 or 3 but no to all the others, you are probably experiencing mild anxiety. The chances are that you're currently experiencing a difficult situation in your life that is causing you stress. Read over our top tips for beating stress on page 63 and try to follow the suggestions. Keep a check on your feelings of anxiety and don't let them escalate to the point where you'd be answering yes to any more of the questions in the checklist. If you've answered yes to questions 4, 5 or 6, it's possible that you're experiencing much more significant anxiety, in which case it is definitely worth you seeing your doctor and asking for advice and

treatment. If you've answered yes to question 7, you've experienced a panic attack. This is a classic symptom of anxiety disorder and if you're not already getting medical treatment, you should see your doctor and ask to be referred to a psychologist or counsellor as soon as possible.

Panic attacks are terrifying experiences in which a person suddenly feels extremely fearful, out of control, out of breath and sometimes even as if they are dying. Often a sufferer won't connect the attack with anxiety as such, but gets caught up in a vicious circle as they then become terrified of experiencing another. Because it's not at all clear what's triggered the initial attack, this can lead some people to avoid social contact and everyday activities. If panic attacks are left untreated, a panic disorder may develop, which can become very disabling. These attacks are one of the most common symptoms of anxiety, but you can still suffer from it without having had one. Whatever form anxiety disorders take, the good news is that psychological treatment has been shown to be up to 90 per cent effective. Speak to your doctor about anti-anxiety medications and a type of psychotherapy called cognitive behavioural therapy, which will give you practical tools for understanding the source of your anxiety and help you deal with it. However, do remember that if you're on the mild end of the anxiety spectrum, it's well worth trying to combat sources of stress actively and factor more relaxation time into your lifestyle before you decide it's time for treatment.

Black and blue

Today, a staggering 120 million people are suffering from depression all over the world. It's by no means just a case of the blues, or even feeling sorry for yourself – instead, it's a very real medical condition that needs proper medical treatment. In fact, if it continues at its current pace, it's estimated that by 2020, depression will be the leading cause of disability and ill-health around the world. When sufferers are in the midst of a depressive episode, they experience one or more of the following symptoms:

- Feelings of sadness and pessimism
- Feelings of being worthless and hopeless
- Loss of interest and pleasure in activities that were once enjoyed
- Decreased energy levels and a sense of being physically slowed down
- An inability to get moving and achieve tasks
- Lack of concentration
- Poor memory
- Difficulty in making decisions
- Difficulty in sleeping, including insomnia, waking up very early in the morning or over-sleeping
- Lack of sex drive
- An affected appetite with subsequent weight loss or gain
- Suicidal thoughts

There are probably several causes for depression. It's known to run in families, particularly a more severe form, bipolar disorder (also known as manic depression), in which, without warning, sufferers swing from extreme highs and manic periods of excess energy to depressive periods as described above. We also know that depression is intrinsically linked with the chemistry of the human brain and, in particular, the way in which our moods and emotions are regulated by chemicals called neurotransmitters.

Serotonin is a neurotransmitter inside your brain that works in much the same way as

Battle of the sexes: when times are tough

- In every country in the world, women are twice as likely to suffer from clinical depression as men. It's believed the difference is due to a gene only women can carry that increases your susceptibility to the condition.

- The gender difference seems to emerge around puberty: before that boys are slightly more likely to get depressed than girls. After the menopause, women's increased susceptibility to depression fades.

- When faced with stress or the blues, men tend to try and distract themselves by seeking out pleasure through sports or partying. Men are more likely than women to reach for alcohol or drugs when the going gets tough.

- Women are more likely to share their problems and seek support from their family or friends. In fact, there's even a name for it: women usually show 'tend or befriend' behaviours when faced with stress, as opposed to men relying more on 'fight or flight'.

- Unfortunately, women also tend to ruminate about things (thinking and talking about a stressful event or situation repeatedly), which underlines feelings of hopelessness and can sometimes even promote depression.

dopamine (see pages 55–6). We know that serotonin's main role is to regulate our moods and it tends to be dysfunctionally low in people suffering from depression, but we don't yet know whether that is a cause or an effect of the illness. Either way, there are all manner of reasons why serotonin can malfunction: too little may be produced in the first place, you might not have enough receptor sites on the receiving cells to pass the whole message along or serotonin may be absorbed by the receiving cells too quickly.

Life's lows

Research has shown that many depressions are triggered by exceptionally stressful life events, such as bereavements or the break-up of important relationships. Think back to your body's stress response and that cocktail of chemicals: we know that continued stress causes elevated levels of the hormone cortisol – over time, this has been shown to lower levels of that vital mood chemical serotonin. It's even thought that surges in cortisol can reduce the number of serotonin receptors in your brain. The stress chemical also wreaks havoc on the parts of your brain that process and produce feelings of pleasure. In particular, the neurotransmitter dopamine (which works across the synapses in your brain in much the same way as serotonin but controls pleasure rather than mood) appears to be stunted when in the presence of very high levels of cortisol, which might partly account for why people suffering from depression struggle to feel pleasure.

The reality is, however, that not everyone experiencing chronic stress or a major trauma will go on to develop depression. Experts now believe that some of us may carry a genetic predisposition to it: if our lives unfold in such a way that we're put under extreme stress or trauma, depression may develop. In a fascinating and unique international study, 847 people born in the 1970s in New Zealand were genetically tested. The research was looking at a gene called 5-HTT, which carries the information for how your brain goes about transporting serotonin. Of course this is by no means the only gene involved in regulating your mood, so there is no such thing as a 'gene for depression'. But this study revealed that 5-HTT does play an important role in your mood. This gene comes in two types: one is short and the other long. You've inherited one copy of it from each of your parents, which means you'll either have two short copies, two long or one of each. After assessing the subjects' life events and incidences of depression, it appears that the long form of the gene carries some sort of protective effect. Those people who had two copies of the short version of the gene were two and a half times more likely to experience depression after a series of stressful events than those who had two long copies. While the precise interaction between genes and life events remains largely uncovered, this is an important step in our understanding of how depression can develop.

Taming depression

If you've never suffered from depression personally or known anyone who has either, you might be tempted to tell a depressed person just to pull themselves together. In a word, don't. For reasons we don't fully understand, depression causes people to be suicidal and if a case is left untreated, this can be a very real risk. Suicide is one of the top ten causes of death around the world; it's even in the top three for people aged 15 to 34. By 2020, it's estimated that 1.5 million people around the world will kill themselves each year. What's more, depression is treatable: there are now a variety of effective anti-depressants available and psychological treatments like cognitive behavioural therapy have been shown to be very useful too. It's not a simple condition to treat and it can take several goes to get the medication that's right and works for you, but nevertheless, if you feel that you or anyone you know is suffering from depression, it's vital you consult a doctor and get further advice and treatment.

For people suffering from moderate or severe clinical depression, medical treatment is the best option. There is no simple checklist of habit-changing, lifestyle-altering advice we can give. However, it's entirely possible to suffer from occasional bouts of mild depression that don't affect you as severely, but still bring you down. In this instance, try taking the steps listed below.

Top tips for coping with depression

- **Talk about it.** Make sure you have a close family member or friend who you can turn to for support and understanding. If you prefer, try calling a depression support group in your local area.

- **Exercise.** Mild to moderate exercise has been proven to improve your mood and is even sometimes used to treat people suffering from milder cases of depression instead of taking tablets.

- **Be patient.** You won't feel better overnight, but improvements in your mood will come gradually. If that in itself fills you with fear, set a time limit for how long you'll wait and see if any improvement comes naturally. If you pass your deadline, make a pact with yourself to talk to your doctor about the depression.

- **Don't make decisions.** If at all possible, try not to make any major life-changing decisions about your job or relationship until the depression has lifted.

- **Spend time with others.** Try not to spend a lot of time on your own as this will only give the negative feelings more of an opportunity to come out. Be around people who like you and want to support you.

- **Don't seek highs.** Alcohol and drugs might bring temporary relief, but they'll swing you low again afterwards.

- **Take it easy.** Don't set yourself huge tasks during this time. Be kind to yourself and don't take on big responsibilities.

- **Don't feel ashamed.** Depression is extremely common nowadays but still carries a stigma. Remind yourself how many people around the world suffer with this condition – you aren't alone. And if things get too much for you, don't delay going to see a doctor straight away.

- **Do whatever feels best.** If you want to try a herbal remedy, such as St John's Wort, there's no reason why you shouldn't, although results are mixed as to how effective it really is. Do be aware though that St John's Wort weakens the effectiveness of the contraceptive pill.

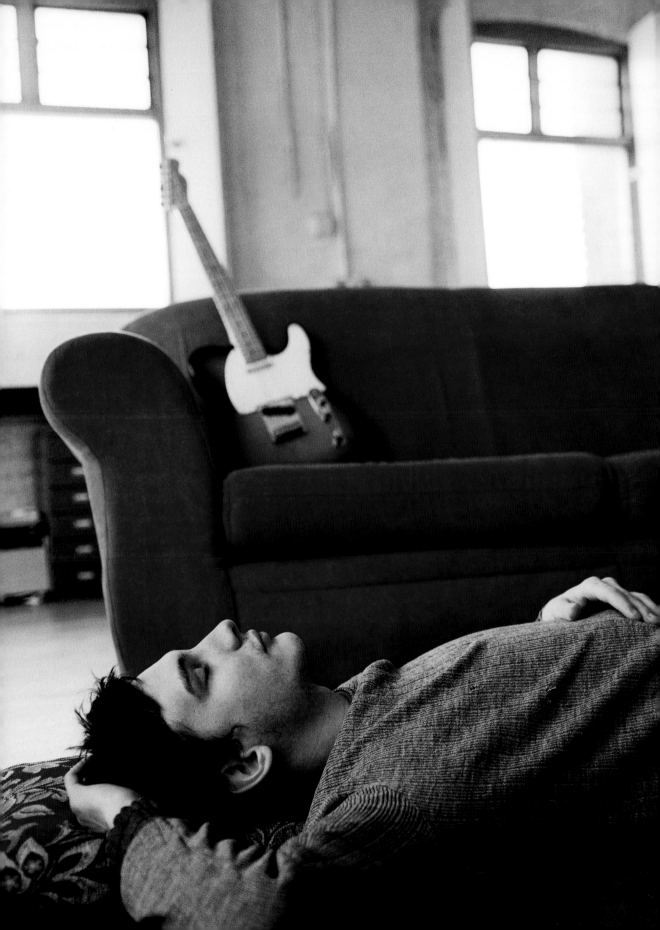

4

Taking Time Out

As evening falls and the stress of your daily grind begins to fade, what's on offer? Increasingly, our culture sees the evening as a time to do all the things we've missed out on during our working hours. If you fancy buying your washing powder at 4 a.m., plenty of supermarkets and shops are now open 24 hours a day; you can chat with someone on the other side of the world at any time on the Internet; many banks and services now offer a round-the-clock telephone facility – you can even hit a nightclub at 6 a.m. for a morning out on the tiles. But as the ubiquitous term '24/7' fast becomes a regular part of our everyday slang, are we missing a trick?

While we might take the view that non-stop access to services, facilities and fun should be everyone's right, our bodies have other plans. When the human body was designed 100,000 years ago, nightfall meant several hours of complete darkness. There wasn't much else to do except sleep and recharge for the coming day's survival chores – hunting down the local sabre-tooth tiger and fixing the occasional salad of seeds and berries.

Like all living things, from bacteria to plants and all other species on the planet, we operate on a daily cycle, and sleep and rest are vital parts of that. In this chapter, we'll be taking a look at what goes on inside you while you're asleep and why depriving yourself of proper rest can have some surprisingly serious consequences. But alas, relaxation isn't fail-safe: when you finally hit the tiredness wall head-on and head off on that two-week break, you'll need to avoid some serious holiday health dangers to make sure you come home feeling fully refreshed.

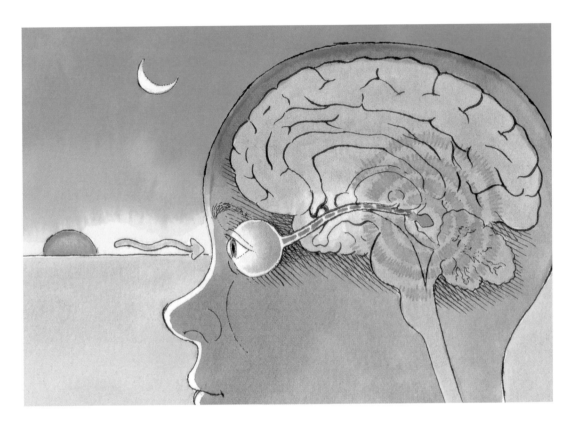

Clocking off

Your body is controlled by approximately 100 complex 'biological clocks', each of which is responsible for regulating different vital functions inside you, such as digestion, temperature, the secretion of hormones, reproduction and growth. Those internal clocks are also known as your circadian rhythms (circadian from the Latin meaning 'around the day'). And remarkably, for reasons we're not yet entirely sure of, your body's clocks all work on a 24-hour timescale.

There's a leader of the pack when it comes to biological timekeeping. That's the master body clock that resides deep within your brain. Here's what happens: information about the current daylight levels around you gets passed from the cells in the retina of your eye through the optic nerve and along to

Above: As daylight falls, messages travel from your eyes to your brain's timekeeper, the SCN (shown here in yellow). It triggers the tiny pineal gland (in blue) to produce the hormone melatonin, which makes you feel sleepy.

the big daddy of circadian rhythms – that's a group of cells called the suprachiasmatic nucleus (SCN) as you'll see in the illustration above. When it comes to keeping time in the vast orchestra of your brain, the SCN is your very own conductor. On top of daylight levels, it also uses clues from your meal times and other social activities to keep track of time. Then, as day and night pass, it broadcasts vital messages across your brain. These messages trigger the production of a cocktail of important chemicals that keep you and your body 'in time'.

We have drift-off

Let's wind back your life to yesterday evening. As the day drew to a close, you were probably unwinding as you watched late-night TV or made the best of that last glass of wine, but it was a different story inside your body. Your SCN had registered that daylight levels had fallen and sent a message to a tiny cone-shaped structure in your brain called the pineal gland. In response, it began pumping out a special sleepiness hormone called melatonin into your bloodstream. As your melatonin levels rose (which normally happens about two hours before bedtime), you started to feel drowsy, your core body temperature dropped and you began to feel ready for sleep.

Once under the covers, most of us take around 20 minutes to drop off and then every 90 minutes or so your brain cycles through five distinct sleep stages. The first two stages are fairly light and you can be woken easily if disturbed. Then, as the electrical activity in your brain is progressively dampened down, complete relaxation takes over and you enter the deeper third and fourth stages. Finally you reach the fifth stage – REM (rapid eye movement) sleep – which occupies a quarter of the night. Your eyes will dart madly back and forth under your eyelids as your brain goes full-tilt into electrical overdrive and begins experiencing highly emotional dreams.

Meanwhile back to last night – deep in your veins, that soporific hormone melatonin probably peaked between around 2 and 4 a.m., insuring that your distinct sleep cycles continued through the night. But while you were hopefully happily exploring the land of nod, there wasn't much rest for your master timekeeper, the SCN. As this morning broke and the light began to rise, it had to be on call to send a wake-up message to another gland in your brain, called the pituitary. As we saw earlier in the section on stress (see page 62), the pituitary gland is part of a complex brain circuit (called the HPA or hypothalamic-pituitary-adrenal axis). A cascade of chemicals gets produced along this path, which ends just above your kidneys at the adrenal glands. Here, adrenaline and cortisol get pumped out – chemicals that raise your heart rate and blood pressure, make you feel alert and help release energy. So, as your cortisol level rose with this morning's light, it put paid to the sleepy effects of last night's melatonin and your brain began to wake up. And just to help you along the way, the pituitary gland did its morning chore as your very own in-built alarm clock – within 30 minutes of first waking, it had triggered a cortisol boost of a massive 100 per cent to ensure you didn't doze off again (in theory, that is, if the well-worn snooze button on most alarm clocks is anything to go by).

How much shuteye is enough?

Scientists have estimated that a century ago, people living in industrialized cities got around nine hours of sleep a night. Nowadays, with our longer working hours and night-time light pollution, the average for city-dwellers is somewhere in the region of less than seven hours. That means you'll spend about 25 years of your life asleep! So is sleep doing its job for you – and what exactly is the point of it in the first place? The early sleep experts wondered whether the behaviour had originally evolved to keep our ancient ancestors out of trouble in the darkness of night on the African savannah. But as people's bedrooms have proved to be relatively safe from roving jungle predators for some time now, that doesn't exactly explain it. Instead, the more likely explanation is that

Case Study
When work gets on top of you

David is 31 and runs his own business dealing with safety systems for trains. It's David's responsibility to make sure everything is working correctly – not a job you'd want to get wrong. 'I constantly feel stressed with my job, it's as if everything rests on your shoulders. I feel really tired but as soon as my head hits the pillow, I can feel my brain going into overdrive. I'll get an idea in the middle of the night and start programming reminders into my mobile phone.' On a bad night, David might only get two hours of sleep. That's making it increasingly hard for him to function during the day. 'Concentration is the main thing. Jobs can take you twice as long and the work you've done is only half as good as what you'd have done on a normal day.'

After taking some advice from a sleep expert, David has recently begun to make some changes to his sleeping pattern. 'Now I'm making a real effort to have a long period of relaxation and do lots of breathing exercises before I even try to get into bed. If I wake up during the night, I do the exercises again and it seems to be working. Even just having one or two better nights of sleep is making a major difference to my stress levels and how I feel about my job.'

Right: Sleep is vital for good reaction times, metabolism and a healthy body and mind.

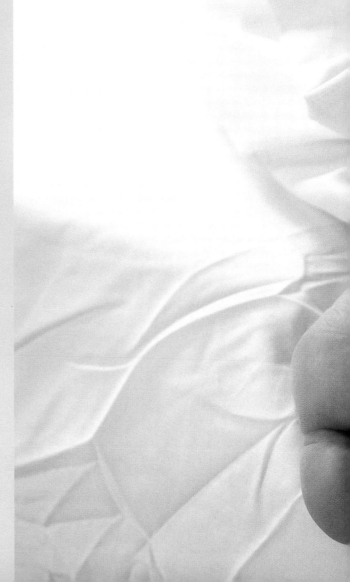

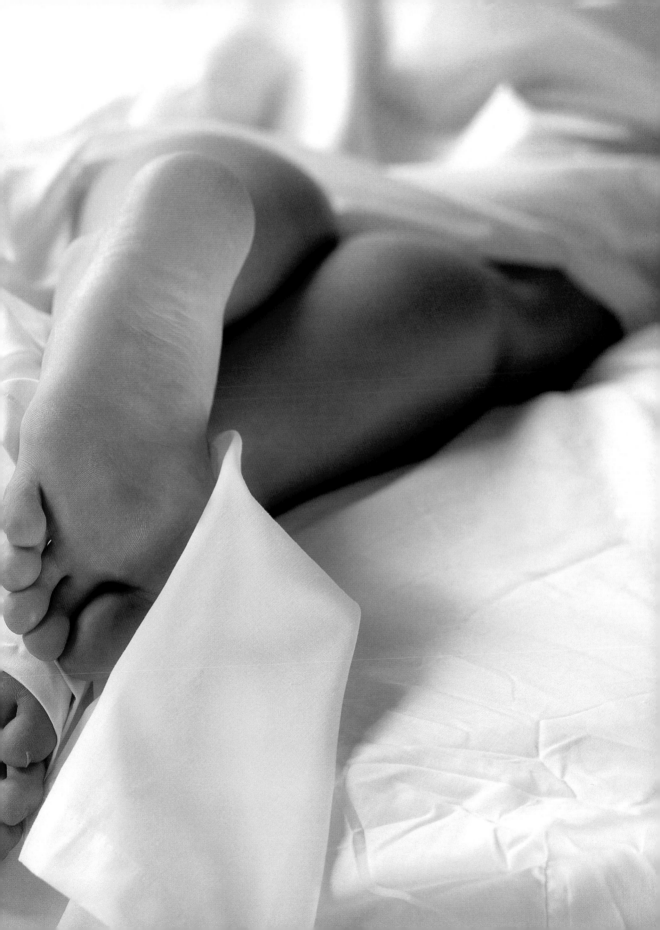

sleep's refreshing and regenerative effects allow various brain, hormonal and growth processes to take place inside you. Essentially, sleep gives your brain and body uninterrupted time to get its biological duster and rubber gloves out and get down to its own special version of internal housekeeping.

While we marvel at the mysterious way sleep does its chores for us, most of the scientific evidence on what exactly those duties are comes from studies in which people have been deprived of their sleep. In 1959, Peter Tripp, a New York City radio DJ, took on a challenge to stay awake continuously for eight days. After four days he started to complain of visual hallucinations, seeing insects, mice and a rabbit running about and also a cabinet drawer catch fire. Nevertheless, he made it and immediately slept for 13 hours straight, emerging unscathed. Six years later, Tripp lost his record to Randy Gardner, a 17-year-old high-school student. Gardner experienced visual problems quite early on and was literally seeing double by the end of his marathon – an astonishing 11 days – quite a feat, when you consider how hideous a mere 36 hours was for John during filming of the sleep episode for BBC3's *Body Hits* series (see page 79)!

Getting into sleep debt

If you think of sleep as time that could be spent more usefully doing something else, what's coming might – ironically enough – be a bit of a wake-up call. Here's what really happens to your body as it gets deprived of sufficient resting time. At first, despite feeling tired after one or several nights of compromised sleeping time, you'll probably be able to carry out most simple tasks relatively well in short bursts. But the real problems begin when major concentration is required. Your judgement will be affected, your social and communication skills will suffer and you'll be far more likely to make bad decisions all round. You might get grumpy and irritable or take unadvisable risks in your daily life, even down to little things like crossing the road against the traffic lights or putting your foot down in the car to get somewhere on time.

Even more worryingly, your attention span and reaction time will be significantly reduced – and if you end up driving when deprived of sleep, there could be serious consequences. In a recent study, a group of men aged 18 to 25 were tested in a driving simulator to compare the effects of alcohol against sleep deprivation. Both drunk drivers and tired drivers were unable to keep up a steady speed or stick to a stable road position, but the most shocking finding came in the figures. Those who hadn't slept for the past 21 hours (not that much if you think about an average late night out) demonstrated equally bad driving skills as those with a blood alcohol measurement of 0.08 per cent. As we saw in Chapter 1, that's the legal limit for driving in most countries around the world. So bear in mind that even an average amount of sleep deprivation – say one or two late nights in a row – could affect your ability as much as being officially 'over the limit'.

While the effects on your mind might be more immediately evident, over time lack of sleep will start to take its toll on your body. Your appetite will increase to compensate for your body's growing need for energy – which obviously could lead to weight gain. On top of that, scientists in the US have shown that people who often get less than six hours' sleep a night seem to have much more sluggish metabolisms. Compared to eight-hours-a-night types, the short-sleepers'

Rate your sleep

1 How long do you take to get to sleep?
Less than 30 minutes = 0 points
Up to 1 hour = 1 point
Up to 2 hours = 2 points
More than 2 hours = 3 points
Your score ☐

2 How many hours of sleep do you usually get?
7 hours or more = 0 points
5 to 6 hours = 1 point
3 to 4 hours = 2 points
2 hours or less = 3 points
Your score ☐

3 How many days each week do you wake up feeling very tired?
None at all = 0 points
1 day only = 1 point
2 to 4 days = 2 points
5 days or more = 3 points
Your score ☐

4 How sleepy do you usually feel at 11 a.m.?
Not at all = 0 points
A little bit = 1 point
Quite a lot = 2 points
A great deal = 3 points
Your score ☐

5 How sleepy do you feel at 3 p.m., having had no alcohol at lunch?
Not at all = 0 points
A little bit sleepy = 1 point
Quite sleepy = 2 points
Very sleepy = 3 points
Your score ☐

6 How sleepy do you feel at 9 p.m., having had no alcohol?
Not at all = 0 points
A little bit sleepy = 1 point
Quite sleepy = 2 points
Very sleepy = 3 points
Your score ☐

Add up your scores and enter your total here ☐

What your score means:
0 to 2 = Your sleep is excellent!

3 to 8 = Your sleep is average, but check out our top tips on page 78 if you want to improve it.

9 to 18 = You have poor quality sleep; try to work on the checklist on page 78 and if there isn't much change after two weeks, see a doctor. It's important to seek medical advice if you experience a strong and ongoing need to sleep – chronic tiredness can be a symptom of such serious medical conditions as depression, anaemia, immune problems and some forms of cancer, although in most cases it's simply due to a big accumulated sleep debt.

Top tips for improving your sleep

• **Ventilate your bedroom and keep it cool.** Your body temperature needs to drop for you to fall asleep.

• **Have an evening hot bath or shower.** But make sure it's only up to an hour before bedtime.

• **Try out a lighter, seasonal duvet.** It's a good idea to stop yourself getting too hot during the night.

• **Keep your bedroom dark.** Light inhibits the production of your sleep hormone, melatonin. Try investing in a thick curtain lining.

• **Take plenty of time getting ready for bed.** This will enable your mind and body to have a good chance to unwind before you try to go to sleep.

• **Monitor your daily caffeine intake.** Avoid any coffee and tea after 9 p.m. Bear in mind that unless herbal tea specifically states it's caffeine-free, it may not be. Carbonated soft drinks, flu remedies and chocolate also contain caffeine, so avoid these just before bedtime.

• **Reduce your weekly alcohol and cigarette intake.** Nicotine is a stimulant, so a cigarette just before bed won't help matters.

• **Don't eat within one or two hours of bedtime.** Eating stimulates your digestive system and metabolism, which means your body will wake up.

• **Do take exercise, but not too near bedtime.**

• **Consider trying out a new mattress and pillow.**

• **Try ear-plugs if your environment is excessively noisy.**

• **Try a relaxation technique.** If you take more than 30 minutes to get off to sleep, try some deep breathing.

• **Don't just lie there.** If you still can't sleep after 30 minutes, get up, do something else and then try again. Lying in bed unable to sleep for ages will induce anxiety.

• **Take a short nap.** If you're so tired during the day that you need to take a nap, limit it to 20 minutes – any longer and you could affect your chances of sleeping that night.

• **Bring your baby to bed.** If you're a new parent and your baby is keeping you awake, you could try bringing your baby into the bed with you during the night. However, make sure the baby sleeps on its back and be cautious about the risk of accidental smothering if you're extremely tired. Studies have also shown that if parents smoke or drink heavily, babies who sleep with them are at increased risk of SIDS (cot death), so bear this in mind.

bodies are only about 60 per cent as efficient at using their hormone insulin to break down glucose (sugars) in the blood into energy. They also need to use a whopping 50 per cent more insulin to carry out that vital metabolic process in the first place. In fact, that's not far off what goes on in your body if you're in the early stages of diabetes.

One possible explanation for this worrying metabolic go-slow can be found in your brain's timekeeping system. Remember the pineal and adrenal glands and the see-saw relationship between their products, the sleep hormone melatonin and the alertness hormone cortisol? If you're regularly not getting enough sleep, your cortisol levels will be raised. In fact, even one night of sleep loss is enough to hike your cortisol levels up by a staggering 45 per cent the following day. To cut a long biological story short, cortisol evolved as part of our ancient and instinctive 'fight or flight' response. In other words, it's part of your body's very own emergency alertness response. As well as being your early morning chemical wake-up call, it also comes out to play whenever you encounter the daily stresses of life, whether that's gridlock at rush hour, an almighty row with your partner or problems at work.

If one of our stone-age ancestors had unexpectedly come up against an angry big beast, it would have made good biological sense for his body to prioritize the processes going on inside him as quickly as it could. He would clearly have needed the alertness, energy and muscular blood supply to run for the hills or fight the predator off, but other bodily functions, such as getting on with the tough job of digesting last night's wildebeest leg, would suddenly have become somewhat less important. So cortisol, combined with the better-known chemical adrenaline, helped

John is deprived of sleep for *Body Hits*

'After a trip to an MOD firing range where I shot pop-up targets with reasonable accuracy, I settled down for my first night of no sleep at the University of Surrey's Sleep Research Centre. Between midnight and 3 a.m. I watched a movie, read a bit, drank a cup of coffee and fiddled with my laptop. I then failed miserably to complete a 3-D replica of Tower Bridge, and chatted with my director until 5 a.m. A couple of hours later, we headed off to a driving simulator. Alarmingly, I was filmed taking a six second nap or 'micro-sleep' at the wheel without even realizing. At 110 km/h (70 mph) on a real motorway, that would have meant I'd gone 125 m (140 yards) fast asleep behind the wheel.'

'By the next evening, I hadn't slept for 36 hours and descended into a very grumpy head space. By 3 a.m. I was all talked out and the urge to kip was unbearable. But at 5.30 a.m., we were back to the firing range to test my decision-making skills. There's no denying that I was more bullish: armed targets got the proper treatment but in the excitement I took out several unarmed civilians as well. It was time to quit before I persuaded them to let me have a go on the tanks! Once home, and contrary to the sleep-deprived celebrities from the past (see page 76), I crashed for hours and then surfaced to encounter three days of jet lag: early morning waking and afternoon sleepiness. Not recommended!'

our ancestors get out of sticky situations, partly by giving them the energy to fight or escape, but also by temporarily switching off functions like the metabolism, the immune system, growth and reproduction so that their bodies could get on with surviving in their 'eat or be eaten' world.

While these days the nearest most of us get to a raw leg of beast is probably in the meat aisle at the supermarket, we're still living with the same set of brain chemicals. So when we get hit by lack of sleep and cortisol levels rise, our immune response and our metabolism will become stunted. Just one night of poor sleep is enough to significantly reduce the action of your special bacteria and virus-killing immune cells. And that intricate mix of lack of sleep, stress and cortisol can unwittingly take you on a rollercoaster of bad all-round health.

When sleep goes bad

Bearing in mind what we now know about the stress hormone cortisol, let's imagine that you're going through a pretty tough time at work or in your relationship. Your cortisol levels will be up. But we also know that cortisol sits firmly on the other end of that see-saw with the sleep hormone, melatonin. So being stressed stops your body's production of melatonin, which can prevent you falling asleep. Meanwhile not sleeping enough can also raise your cortisol further, making you even more stressed. It's the core of a particularly nasty vicious circle. One in four people now complains of insomnia – and for a number of different reasons.

Being physically unable to sleep well (or when you want to) for whatever reason wreaks havoc on your body. Millions of people around the world suffer and you can imagine how much that hikes up national health bills. We've seen how even one or two nights of bad sleep can affect the workings of your mind and body, but if your sleep 'debt' mounts up day after day, you could be in for big trouble. Complete our specially designed sleep questionnaire on page 77 to find out whether your sleeping pattern could be setting you up for health problems.

Time out

As well as making adjustments to our sleeping environment and behaviour before bedtime, we also need to find ways of including more relaxation in our lives generally. Set aside more time for sleep and rests if you can. If you're the kind of person who actively enjoys yoga, pilates or the occasional massage, the chances are your sleep and energy levels are probably pretty good. But for most of us, hectic schedules don't always permit such treats. Instead, we rely on an annual vacation to pay off our accumulated sleep debts. Sleeping for just two extra hours each night for a fortnight can neatly erase 30 hours of sleep loss. Combine that with the all-round relaxation of a change of scene, climate and a break from work and other chores and a holiday looks like the ideal way to break your stress-fatigue cycle. But beware, travelling abroad also presents its very own health risks and, believe it or not, they start just as soon as you get on the plane.

Come fly with me

You've made it to the airport on time, remembered your passport, the sun cream and those novels you've been trying to read for the last six months. But as you finally sink into your seat and start looking forward to arriving at your holiday destination, your body's about to hit a wall of physiological challenges.

If airlines simply pumped in the fresh air from outside the plane at 9000 m (30,000 feet) up, it'd be far too thin and wouldn't contain enough oxygen to keep everyone inside alive. But if they just recycled the same air inside the cabin all the way to your holiday haven, there wouldn't be enough oxygen in that air either, especially on a long-haul flight. So the solution is to recycle a proportion of the air throughout the journey and mix it with some of the thin fresh air from outside the plane (usually about a 50/50 mix). But, surprisingly, the pressure of that air mixture is still the equivalent of suddenly finding yourself at an altitude of 2500 m (8000 feet) up. In fact, the air inside most planes is thinner and drier than it is in the Sahara desert, which explains the unpleasant feeling of dryness we all associate with flying. Unfortunately, this discomfort can be more than skin deep.

Dehydration is a serious air travel hazard because it makes your blood thicker, slowing down its flow around your body. And if you also factor in those salty pre-dinner snacks, the free alcoholic drinks and sedentary movie-watching followed by sporadic, uncomfortable periods of sleep, there could be trouble ahead.

What is Deep Vein Thrombosis?

In the course of a normal day, the chances are you'll move around quite a lot. The concentration of your blood cells will be kept under control, although tiny clots may form

Top anti-DVT tips

● **Drink plenty of water.** Drinking water before you get on the plane and during the journey can increase your blood flow by about 5 per cent.

● **Avoid alcohol, salty food and caffeine.** These all increase dehydration.

● **Move around on the flight.** The risk of DVT isn't so much to do with how much leg room the airline gives you, but more about how mobile you are during the flight. Try the following two simple exercises:
1 Bend and straighten your legs, toes and feet every half an hour or so.
2 Press the balls of your feet down hard on the floor to increase blood flow in your legs.

● **Avoid knocking yourself out with sleeping pills.** You'll be immobile for too long.

● **Invest in a pair of flight socks.** These are tight elastic knee-high stockings that put pressure on the blood vessels in your legs, pushing the blood up to your heart and keeping the flow moving.

● **Or take aspirin.** These cost just 2p a tablet and thin your blood, making the formation of clots less likely. Check first with your doctor that it's all right for you to take them as some people have a rare allergy. All being well, take half a tablet the day before you fly, before the journey itself and the day after.

● **If you are concerned, seek your doctor's advice.** If you do experience any pain or swelling in your legs (especially in one more than the other), or if you have breathing difficulties up to two weeks after you fly, consult your doctor immediately.

occasionally. With all your daily activity, any clots should easily get knocked apart and never cause a problem. But if you're dehydrated, your blood becomes thicker and it's much easier for your blood cells to get into a 'traffic jam', creating a more serious clot. So just being on a plane with all that dry air is putting you at risk of blood clots. Add in the effects of all that immobility over several hours and there's an even greater chance that clots won't be dispersed by blood flow.

Deep Vein Thrombosis (DVT) is a condition in which blood clots form in the deep veins of the legs. It causes pain, swelling, tenderness and possibly even redness, usually at the back of one of your legs below the knee. But the real problems begin if that clot manages to work its way up to your lungs. There it can block your circulation and that can be fatal. A recent study showed that one in 100 long-haul travellers went on to develop potentially dangerous blood clots as a result of their journey. However, two-thirds of these already had medical conditions that made a clot more likely, so don't get overly anxious about it, but do know your facts – use our risk assessment below and top tips on page 81.

Check whether any of the main risk factors for DVT apply to you:

1 Have you had a previous history of blood clots, circulation problems or a stroke? YES/NO

Top tips for beating jet lag

● **If flying east, book a night flight.** It's best to arrive the following day in the late afternoon or early evening.

● **If flying west, take a lunchtime flight.** Go for a flight that will touch down in your destination in the late afternoon.

● **Start adjusting to the local routine.** As soon as you board the plane reset your watch to the local time at your destination.

● **Have an early night.** When you arrive at your destination, get out and have a meal, maybe a drink or two, but go to bed early.

● **Try a melatonin pill.** If you've crossed five or more time zones, consider taking a synthetic melatonin pill for the first three nights of your holiday (unless you are pregnant, breast-feeding or suffer from asthma). These pills can be bought from health food shops in the US (where it's treated as a food supplement) or on the Internet, but are not currently available in the UK. Scientists have found that taking a dose close to bedtime helps to make you feel sleepy, thus reducing jet lag symptoms. Similarly, on your return, a dose of melatonin taken at bedtime for the first three nights may speed up your body's readjustment to the new time zone.

● **Fly home overnight.** When returning home, from either direction, opt for a night flight that arrives early the next morning and avoid work for the rest of the day if possible.

● **Have a nap.** If you feel wiped out on your return, sleep for an hour; don't kill yourself staying awake until bedtime.

2 Does anyone in your family have a tendency to blood problems? YES/NO

3 Are you currently undergoing cancer treatment? YES/NO

4 Have you recently had a general anaesthetic for an operation? YES/NO

5 Are you a smoker? YES/NO

6 Are you over 40? YES/NO

7 Are you pregnant or have you recently had a baby? YES/NO

8 Do you take the contraceptive pill or hormone replacement therapy (HRT)? YES/NO

If you answered yes to any of the above questions, your risk of DVT is higher than average. Whenever you fly, you should follow our tips for minimizing the risk. If you answered yes to any of the risk factors 1 to 4, you should consult your doctor before you set off on your trip.

Lagging behind

So you've made it through jet travel unscathed. But the further you've flown, the more likely you are to encounter a body-boggling trauma on arrival. Think body-clock hell, otherwise known as jet lag.

As we saw in the earlier section on sleep (pages 72–80), your mind and body are kept in time thanks to your master body-clock, the SCN (or suprachiasmatic nucleus). But way back when your SCN was originally designed, flying across thousands of kilometres in a matter of mere hours wasn't exactly an option for your average caveman. Once again, technology has overtaken the human body. The SCN simply can't adapt to a new far-flung time zone as quickly as you can travel there. So while it's busy playing catch-up, your entire body will be out of sync with the local environment. You'll experience sleepiness during the day, be wide awake at 3 a.m., feel like you've got the IQ of a fence post and fancy your meals at very odd hours indeed.

Although the SCN is your brain's time supervisor, scientists believe that each of the many biological clocks inside you must adapt to a new time zone at its own rate. So while you try to relax and enjoy the start of your holiday, there's timekeeping mayhem going on inside you. Worse still, even though you tend to get over these symptoms in two to three days, they're all set to sting you again on your return home.

So if you've picked an exotic holiday destination that involves crossing a handful of time zones, what can you do to help your body adjust as quickly as possible? Check out our top tips (see opposite) for beating the lag.

Here comes the sun

There's nothing better than stretching out in the warming heat of the golden sun and lapping up the rays on your holiday. But while sunshine improves your mood, helps you relax and is part and parcel of most people's holidays, it poses serious risks to your health.

Take a look at a close-up view of your skin (see page 84). Depending on your size, your skin measures around 2 square metres (22 square feet) and weighs an incredible 3.2 kg (7 lb). It's made up of some 300 million special skin cells. The unique colour of your skin is determined by the skin's pigment, melanin, which is found in the epidermis or upper layer of your skin tissue. Tiny granules of the pigment are produced in special cells called melanocytes. Amazingly, whether you're an African bushman or someone born in the north of Scotland, you're likely to have exactly the same number of melanocytes in your skin – between 1000 and 2000 per square centimetre (0.15 square inch) to be precise. In darker-skinned people, those melanocytes are just a whole lot busier producing much bigger granules of melanin.

So why does your skin make melanin in the first place? Well, to put it simply, the sun is staggeringly powerful. In just 15 minutes, it can radiate as much energy around the planet as the world's population consumes in coal, oil, gas, etc., over the course of a whole year. But that energy comes in the form of ultraviolet rays (three types: UVA, UVB and UVC) and those are potentially harmful to our bodies. Most scientists believe that our ancestors who lived in places where they got full-on solar radiation, for example the tropics of Africa, Asia and Australia, were designed to have darkly pigmented skin to give them extra protection, while those living in areas

where there wasn't so much sun, for example, Northern Europe, ended up with much lighter skins. Of course, that biological solution couldn't really take into consideration two-week breaks spent frying our bodies on a Mediterranean beach – which is where the problems start for light-skinned people.

So, as you're sprawled out on a gorgeous beach, soaking up the sun, what's going on in your skin? As soon as the UV hits your epidermis, your melanocytes go into emergency overdrive, producing much more

Below: The sun's ultraviolet rays trigger cells in your skin called melanocytes to produce more of the natural pigment melanin. You might think the results look good, but tanning is your skin's emergency reaction to ultraviolet damage.

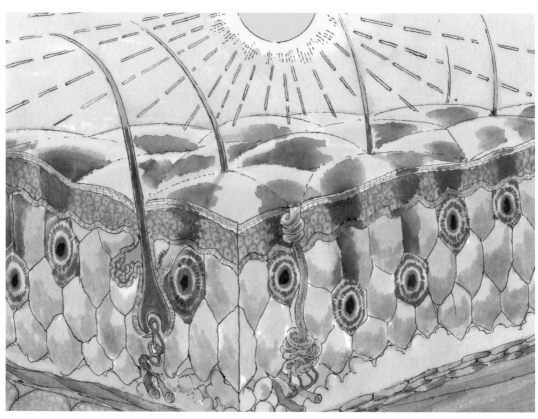

melanin in a drastic attempt to protect your skin from further UV damage. What that really means is that while you're admiring your newly bronzed tone, you body's alarm bells are ringing. The fact is that if you've got light skin, you'll only start to tan once the UV rays have already reached the bottom layer of your epidermis – by which time UV damage will already have taken place.

The damage starts as the UV destroys your skin's connective tissues, collagen and elastin, which with time will cause wrinkling and sagging – in other words, premature ageing. More seriously, UV causes your body to produce dangerous chemicals called free radicals, which can actually damage the DNA inside your skin cells and lead to cancer.

The lobster look

If you're light-skinned, the chances are you've been there at one time or another – just half an hour too long lying by the pool, or an accidental nap on the beach, and before you knew it you were positively pink. Interestingly, sun burn isn't the same thing as a heat burn. At the first sign of UV damage, your immune system leaps into action, pumping out a cocktail of chemicals to start the clean-up operation. Because your body needs to get those emergency services to where they're needed pretty damn quick, your blood flow gets hugely increased, making the skin inflamed and red. It's painful, embarrassing and what's more very dangerous. Shockingly, getting badly sunburnt can double your risk of developing skin cancer.

When moles turn nasty

Your moles are areas of your skin in which those pigment-producing cells, the melanocytes, are most densely packed. And because your melanocytes are where UV hits

hardest, your moles are most susceptible to damage. If some of the DNA in a mole gets mutated by the UV, a rogue cell is created that duplicates itself out of control, making a cancerous tumour. Last year, 60,000 people in the UK were diagnosed with skin cancer and cases of malignant melanoma have doubled in the last ten years. It's vital you keep an eye on all your moles and birthmarks, if you have any. Don't forget you probably have some on your back, which you might not be able to see easily, so ask a friend or partner to check those from time to time. Here's what you need to watch out for:

● Has the mole changed in size? YES/NO
● Has it got darker or changed colour in any way? YES/NO
● Does the mole have an uneven outline? YES/NO
● Is its colour uneven? YES/NO
● Does it ever itch, feel tender or hurt in any way? YES/NO
● Has it ever bled? YES/NO

If you answered yes to any of the questions above, you need to consult your doctor without delay. Don't panic as these symptoms don't necessarily mean you have skin cancer, but it does need to be ruled out straight away. The bottom line is that if you do develop skin cancer, getting treatment as early as possible could save your life. If you answered no to all of the questions, keep them in mind and look out for any changes in your moles over time.

Holiday bellies

One of the joys of going away on holiday is trying out new and unusual food. But unfortunately, 50 per cent of all British holidaymakers travelling abroad also get to try

The truth about you and the sun

Despite the dangers of the sun, we all know that having a tan makes you feel and look better, in the short term at least. So how safely are you striking the balance between enjoying your holidays and saving your skin? Take our test to find out – see how many of the statements below apply to you, then check out the facts below:

1 **Going on a sunbed before my holiday will help me to build up a tan safely before I get to my destination.**
YES/NO

2 **I always use sun protection creams when I lie out in the sun so I'm not at risk.**
YES/NO

3 **I only spend a few weeks a year in the sun so I should be fine.**
YES/NO

4 **When I'm on holiday I don't lie out at midday because that's the most dangerous time of day for strong sun.**
YES/NO

5 **When you've built up a base tan, it's safe to start using less sun cream or cream with a lower SPF (sun protection factor) rating.**
YES/NO

6 **If you want to be really safe and bronzed, the best way is to use a fake tan lotion.**
YES/NO

Check our answers to see how you fared:
1 Don't be fooled that sunbeds are safe. They produce UV rays just like the sun but you don't tend to use sun protection creams when you use one, making them very dangerous indeed. Also, each machine varies in the amount of UV (mostly UVA) it pumps out so it's hard to be sure exactly how much UV exposure you're getting.

2 It's true that using SPF creams does minimize the risk of sun damage but do bear in mind these sun cream tips:
– Don't even bother buying cream that's below SPF 15 – and you should really consider using one that's at least SPF 25.
– Make sure the lotion you buy says it protects against both UVA and UVB radiation – not all of them do.
– Apply the cream thickly at least 30 minutes before you go out into the sun. This is vital for it to protect you properly.
– Always remember to reapply the cream after you go for a swim.
– Don't only rely on SPF lotion. Take a sunhat, sunglasses and a shirt or sarong to cover up with as well.

3 Two weeks a year in the sun might not sound like much but that's not necessarily the case. In fact, a fortnight spent basking in Mediterranean summer rays is the equivalent of a whole year's worth of UK sun exposure – intensely packed into 14 days to put your skin under even more stress.

4 It's true that midday tends to be the most dangerous time for UV exposure as the sun is at its highest point. But that's the peak of a much longer period between 11 a.m. and 3 p.m. when the sun is very strong. Try to avoid lying out in the sun during those times – that's when most skin damage will occur. That doesn't mean you have to be holed up indoors – just choose to relax in the shade instead.

5 Don't forget that any sign of a tan means that UV damage has already occurred in your skin. Although we all tend to think of being tanned as something positive and healthy, try to change your mindset and start connecting tanning with danger.

6 It's true that fake tan lotions are the safest way to be bronzed, but just because you're browner doesn't mean that you're also more protected from sun burn and damage. If possible use a fake tanner that has an SPF included or, if not, don't forget to slap on the sun lotion on top of your fake tan.

out a nasty dose of diarrhoea. Follow our top tips to make sure you don't end up spending your hard-earned break in your hotel bathroom:

- Drink bottled water. Make sure the seal on any bottle you buy is intact as in some countries street sellers simply refill bottles with tap water. Remember to avoid ice in drinks too.
- Avoid salad and unpeeled raw fruit and vegetables – they may have been washed in local water.
- Pay attention to the temperature of the food you're eating. If it's meant to be cold, make sure it's really cold – that means it's been properly stored and prepared. If it's cooked, it needs to be piping hot. Don't be fooled by appearances either: you're far more likely to get ill eating food from a luke-warm buffet in a smart five-star hotel than from a freshly cooked meal served up at a simple street stall.
- Avoid seafood.
- If you're in a high-risk country, avoid any food that hasn't been cooked, boiled or peeled, especially when eating in restaurants.
- Avoid ice cream and milk.
- A recent survey showed that one in five ice cubes in foreign holiday resorts is contaminated with bacteria from faeces. Don't assume foreign hygiene standards will match your own.
- If you do get ill, try to avoid taking anti-diarrhoea medicines unless it's very severe and you can't find a doctor. Generally, these medicines work by bunging you up, which can hinder your body's own attempts to get rid of the bug. Often it's a case of better out than in. But be sure to drink plenty of water or use oral rehydration powders as diarrhoea causes extreme dehydration. If you get a severe bout, try to see a local doctor first to get prescription medication.

Holiday health checklist

When you're next preparing to jet off to an exotic foreign destination, use our checklist for what you'll need to take with you to stay healthy while you're away.

- **Medical and travel insurance** – don't even think about leaving the country without it. If you're a British citizen travelling within the EU, pick up an E111 form from any post office. If you're heading outside the EU, ask your travel agent for advice on how to get insurance.

- **Vaccinations** – these vary depending on what country you're travelling to so check out requirements well in advance.

- **Anti-malaria medication** – ask your doctor or pharmacist, use an up-to-date guidebook or contact MASTA, the travellers' health organization (see page 170 for details), to find out whether you need to take anti-malaria pills.

- **Flight socks or aspirin tablets** – the aspirin comes in handy not only to protect against DVT but as a good all-round painkiller should you need one on holiday.

- **Melatonin pills** (see page 82)

- **Sun tan lotions** (preferably SPF 25 and protecting against UVA and UVB radiation)

- **Anti-diarrhoea tablets** – use for severe bouts only when you can't get to see a doctor.

- **Oral rehydration powders** – if you start vomiting, get diarrhoea or simply get dehydrated in hot weather, use these to balance your water and salt levels quickly.

- **Condoms** – whether you're single or travelling with your long-term partner, these are vital. It's worth taking some with you even if you're on the contraceptive pill. If you get sick with vomiting or diarrhoea, you won't get the pill's usual protection and you'll have to use another contraceptive for seven days after you've recovered. Check your pill information leaflet for instructions before you go.

- **Hydrocortisone cream** – this is available over the counter and is useful for insect bites and other minor skin irritations.

- **Antiseptic cream** – for any cuts or bites that get nasty.

- **Non-drowsy anti-histamine tablets** – if you get covered in mosquito bites, taking one of these is the fastest way of getting rid of the itching and discomfort.

- **Insect repellent** – if you're going to an area where mosquitos are rife, buy one that contains as much of the chemical DEET as possible. You might want to consider taking coils and plug-in devices too, and a mosquito net to protect you during the night.

- **Basic first aid** – scissors, bandages, plasters, tweezers, thermometer. If you're going into remote areas, you should consider taking a special traveller's health pack containing syringes.

- **Antibiotics** – if you're travelling to distant climes for a long period of time, you might want to ask your doctor for a course of broad spectrum antibiotics to keep with you should you develop anything nasty.

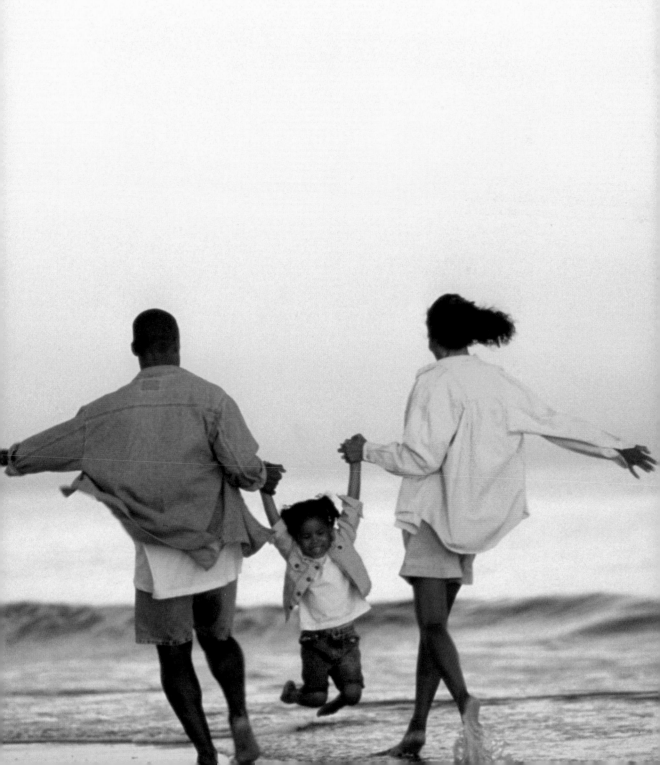

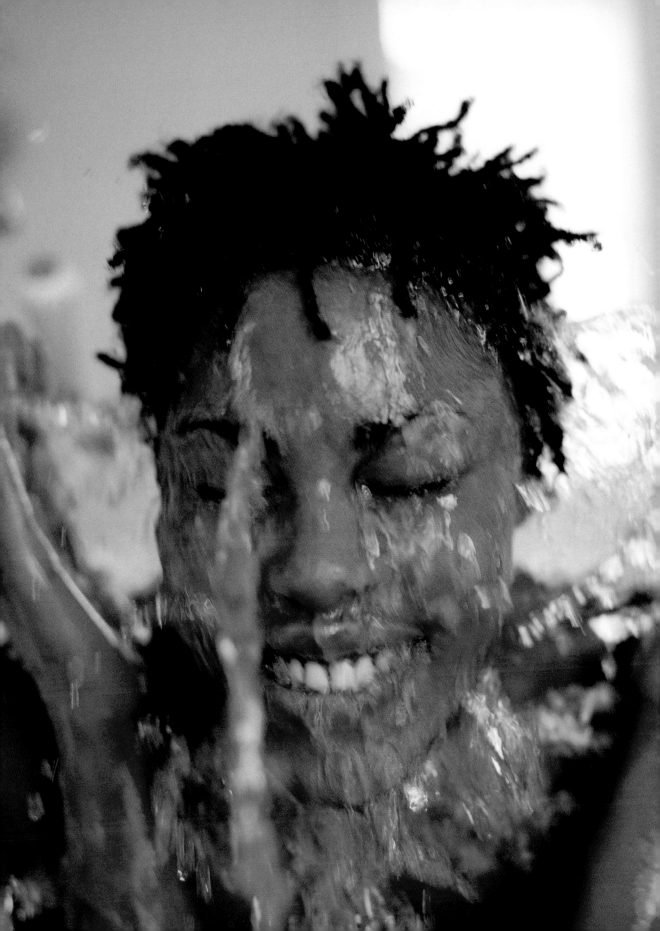

5

Looking Good

When you look in the mirror, what leaps to your eye first – a volcanic-sized pimple, a receding hairline or a road map of wrinkles? Could you even bear to examine your entire naked body in a mirror? For the vast majority of us, how we look really does matter – and it's not just down to pure vanity. Studies show that when someone meets you, they make instant, almost unconscious judgements about your attractiveness in under a second – and those opinions usually stick. What's more, research has revealed that people who are more attractive tend to have more friends and find better jobs and more attractive partners – they even get treated more leniently if they ever end up in court. While culture and fashion obviously play a part, judging attractiveness seems to be an intrinsic part of our psychological fabric. Even a three-month-old baby will spend longer gazing at photographs of attractive faces than those of average-looking ones. Whether it's facial symmetry, a well-proportioned body or clear glowing skin, looking good is really all about what your genes have to offer: across cultures, beauty reflects an intricate and complex mix of symbols of health and fertility.

In our world the quest for beauty is tireless. You can have chemicals injected into your face to hold back the ravages of time, get individual follicles of hair moved from one part of your scalp to another to fight hair loss, or even go under the knife to permanently alter parts of your body. And such options are no longer only the domain of rich film stars or celebrities. In this chapter, we'll get to the bottom of the most common everyday grooming concerns – spots, wrinkles, body odour and hair loss – exploding some long-standing myths along the way. We'll also show you how learning to love the skin you're in can do wonders for your overall happiness and wellbeing.

Skin deep

You probably first thought about your skin's condition as you became a teenager. As hormone levels increase rapidly during puberty, the body can become overly sensitive to the male hormone testosterone (women also produce tiny amounts of this). That means occasional spots, pimples, whiteheads, blackheads and, in more severe cases, acne. But for many, spots aren't only restricted to the teenage years: in fact, some people experience outbreaks well into adulthood. Acne is the most common skin disease in the world and it's estimated that almost 85 per cent of us experience it at some point in our lives.

Let's take a single spot: why does it appear in the first place? As you'll see in the illustration below, your skin contains special sebaceous glands that produce an oily substance called sebum. It's thought that this helps to make the skin waterproof while also keeping it comfortably lubricated. If a sebaceous gland in your skin pumps out a bit too much sebum, it can make the nearby hair follicle overly oily. If the same follicle also happens to have a lot of dead skin cells in it, they'll block the sebum from making its way up and out on to the surface of your skin. Instead it builds up around the follicle, making a blackhead. If bacteria (which are naturally present on the surface of your skin) get into that skin pore, the oil builds up even further around the hair and gets infected. That's when you'll see redness. Pus builds up

Below: Under the red, inflamed surface of the skin, tiny hair follicles can become blocked with bacteria, sebum and pus. A pustule must form and burst to relieve the pressure and free the sebum.

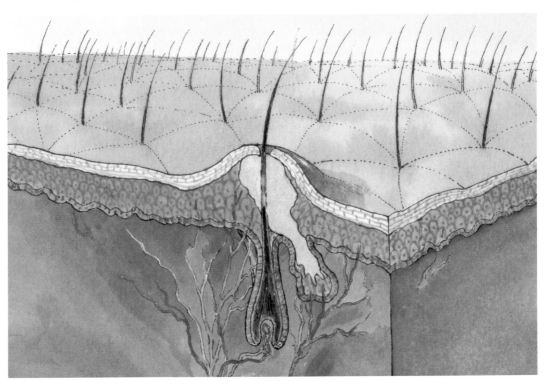

Spot the myths

Answer the following statements:

1 Spots can be caused by eating too much chocolate or fried food.
TRUE/FALSE

2 Spots mean your skin is dirty so you should try washing it more often.
TRUE/FALSE

3 Covering spots in make-up only makes matters worse.
TRUE/FALSE

4 You should never squeeze or pick a spot.
TRUE/FALSE

5 Lying out in the sun clears up spots.
TRUE/FALSE

6 Unless you've got severe acne, there's no need to go to a doctor.
TRUE/FALSE

Now check out how you fared:
1 FALSE. One of the oldest myths about spots is that they're caused by too much sugar or fat in your diet. In fact, studies have shown that there's absolutely no link between chocolate or fatty foods and spots.

2 FALSE. Dirt doesn't cause spots. The bacteria that infect a blocked skin pore, turning it into a spot, are usually harmless and live all over your skin. It's your sebaceous glands producing too much sebum or oil that are to blame. Excessive washing can cause your skin to dry out, which won't help matters as the excess oil starts beneath the surface – instead, all that cleansing will just irritate your skin further.

3 FALSE. Make-up can't cause spots (unless you get a rare allergic reaction to a product). When it comes to spot-prone skin, make-up should help to improve your confidence and as long as you use oil-free or non-comedogenic (non-pore-clogging) products – check the label – and wash them off each night, there should be no problem.

4 FALSE. Generations of mothers have pleaded with their pimply kids not to pick at their spots. In fact, as long as you follow our advice on page 94 on how and when to do it properly, there should be no problem.

5 FALSE. It's been widely shown that while lying out in the sun might appear to bring temporary relief from spots by drying the skin out, it's not an effective treatment and it also means you're exposing yourself to the sun's potentially harmful ultraviolet rays, which can cause sunburn, premature ageing and skin cancer (see pages 83–5).

6 FALSE. Don't suffer in silence: if you've been plagued by regular spots for some time now and have found that over-the-counter remedies aren't working, it's worth getting some specialist advice from your doctor or a dermatologist (see our top tips on pages 94–5 on what treatments you can expect). You could be saving yourself from long-term scarring.

Top tips for clear skin

- **To squeeze or not to squeeze?**
Whether you've got one spot or a hundred, the same rules apply. If the spot consists of a red raised area only, try your best not to touch, pick or squeeze it; at this stage, any intervention from your fingers – or worse still, your fingernails – may just push the infection deeper into your skin, making matters much worse. Once a white or yellowish pustule or head has appeared, the time to squeeze has arrived. First wash and dry your hands thoroughly: you have all sorts of bacteria on your hands and you don't want to infect the spot further with them. Take a tissue and cover each of your squeezing fingers with it – this should protect your skin from whatever nasties are in the pustule. Carefully pop the head off the spot but if you see clear fluid or blood coming out, stop immediately. Further picking or squeezing will simply cause damage to the skin tissue and mean it will take longer to heal. Wash and dry your hands again and apply an antiseptic or a drop of tea-tree oil to the spot. Getting rid of a pustule like this will help the spot heal quicker than if you left it to its own devices, but don't be tempted to break the rules above as you'll be left with more of a mess than when you started.

- **Avoid oily creams.** Some face creams and make-up products contain oils. If you've already got spots or are prone to them, oily beauty products could exacerbate the problem so be sure to buy products that are oil-free or non-comedogenic. The same goes for sun protection creams that are particularly oil-rich. Remember that spots don't only appear on your face, so if you find them appearing on your back or chest, they could be triggered by oily moisturizers or sun creams. Some hair products such as waxes, gels and de-frizzers can also trigger spots, particularly around your hairline.

- **Eliminate bacteria.** Remember that bacteria can breed on make-up sponges, brushes, puffs and applicators. Be sure to give them a regular wash in hot water with a little washing-up or handwashing liquid. Leave them out to dry properly before you use them again.

- **Watch out for sweat.** Getting hot and sweaty can make spots worse. If you exercise regularly or play sport, try to wear clothing that is mostly cotton to allow skin to breathe. Synthetic fabrics such as nylon and polyester can increase heat and sweat when you're wearing them during sport or exercise. Make sure you wash thoroughly as soon as possible afterwards.

- **Visit your pharmacy.** If you've got mild acne or even just the occasional spot, you could try various over-the-counter remedies. These lotions and creams usually contain benzyl peroxide or salicylic acid, which work by drying out the skin and clearing the blocked pores. Both these ingredients are powerful and available in a variety of strengths – don't start with the strongest as it may cause irritation and redness. Try the weakest first and be patient. If there's no improvement after a while, try a stronger variety. If you'd rather stick to natural products, you could try dabbing a bit of undiluted tea-tree oil on to your spots.

- **See the doctor.** If those over-the-counter remedies haven't made any difference after a couple of months, make an appointment with your doctor. The first line of treatment will probably be a course of antibiotics. This could be a topical gel or lotion, which you'll apply directly on to your skin, or tablets which you'll need to take every day. Antibiotics work by killing the bacteria that cause spots in the first place. Different types work for different people. If you haven't seen much improvement after a couple of months, ask your doctor about trying a different type of treatment. If you're female, the doctor might get you to try a particular type of contraceptive pill that contains an anti-androgen and can sometimes help acne. Bear in mind that other types of contraceptive pill can sometimes exacerbate spots, so you might want to try switching brands.

● **Consult a dermatologist.** If you're not happy with the treatment you're getting from your doctor, you should ask to be referred to a skin specialist, who will have much more experience treating such conditions. One of the treatments available to those with more severe acne is a drug called isotretinoin (known as Roaccutane in the UK or Accutane in the US). This works by 'switching off' the sebaceous glands. It's very effective and prevents acne recurring in nearly 80 per cent of cases. However, there can be serious side-effects including liver problems and extreme birth defects should you get pregnant while on the drug. Some patients have reported suffering depression after taking it too. It's best used for very severe cases of acne only and patients must be closely monitored by a doctor while they're taking the tablets (a course of the drug is normally a few months).

● **Get support.** If your spots are really getting you down, talk to your doctor about it. Treatment can take a while to get right, but do persevere and consider contacting a local acne support group (see page 170) if you're feeling low about it.

● **Treat scars.** If you've had spots or acne in the past that have healed up or been treated successfully, the chances are you may have some scarring or pockmarks. There are chemical peels and laser treatments available that can reduce these, if they bother you. Ask a dermatologist for advice on what treatment might work best for you.

behind the blockage and the sebaceous gland in question will get inflamed and sore. Finally, a pustule will form and the pressure of the build-up of pus will force the nasty stuff out of the pore.

If you suffer from acne, your body's reaction to your testosterone means that it will tip many of your sebaceous glands into producing far too much sebum, leaving you highly prone to developing large angry spots. This can occur in the pores all over the face, neck, shoulders, chest or back. Each pore can become a spot, so considering you've got 900 pores in each square centimetre of your face, you can imagine just how bad acne can get. Dermatologists rate the condition as being mild, moderate or severe. If you suffer from the occasional spot, it's very unlikely to be classed as acne. However, regular spots in a particular area indicate that you might be at the mild end of the spectrum. People with more severe acne are likely to be constantly plagued with spots and might even develop large inflamed lumps and cysts. Spots cause people an enormous amount of misery and can have a huge effect on their confidence and self-esteem. On top of that, even mild to moderate acne can cause long-term or permanent scarring. Try taking our test on page 93, then follow our top tips on pages 94–5 to find out how best to treat spots yourself and when to seek medical advice.

Wrinkle wars

No-one wants to look old. Your skin is one of the first features to show age – as the years go by, its elasticity and smoothness diminish. If you gently pinch the skin on the back of a young child's hand and then let it go, you'll see that it returns to its place quickly and easily. Now try the same test on an 80 year old and the skin will take significantly longer to fall back into place.

Your skin's elasticity is down to substances called collagen and elastin. As you can see in the illustration opposite, with age your body's supplies of collagen break down, the skin becomes less supple and elastic and, as a result, wrinkles start to form. While the rate at which you age is probably largely governed by your genes, two lifestyle factors also have a huge part to play in our war against wrinkles.

If you're a smoker or a sun-worshipper, your skin will age significantly faster than it otherwise would. Cigarette smoke and the sun's harmful ultraviolet rays both trigger the production of high levels of enzymes that destroy your skin's collagen. In a recent US study, scientists got to the bottom of how the sun can damage the skin by asking a group of subjects to bare their buttocks to a single mild dose of UVB rays, which are one of the three different types of ultraviolet rays the sun produces – UVB is believed to be responsible for sunburn and the DNA damage in our cells that can lead to skin cancer. In the case of this study, the dose was just enough to cause slight skin reddening (in other words, far less than would trigger proper sunburn). The researchers then analyzed skin samples from the test area of the buttocks and also from an area beside it that hadn't been exposed to the UV rays. Less than one day after exposing the subjects to the rays, the test areas of skin revealed four-fold increases in three different types of enzymes that destroy both collagen and elastin. You can imagine how long days spent lying on the beach might affect your skin, or continual everyday exposure to the sun's UV rays over many years spent in a hot country.

Don't be fooled by what you see when you look in the mirror. You might not be old enough for wrinkles to have really set in yet, but take a look at the two photographs on page 98. The first image shows a young woman as you might see her with your naked eye. Her skin appears to be in good condition, give or take a few freckles. However, the second photograph has been taken by a dermatologist using a special camera with an ultraviolet light. It shows up the UV damage just under the surface of the woman's skin, which can't be seen with the naked eye. The more sun you've been exposed to over the years, the more dark patches would show up on this type of photograph. Remember that freckles and tans are your body's ways of reacting to the sun's UV damage as it takes place in your skin – and in the long term that not only means you're at increased risk of developing skin cancer but also that your skin will age prematurely. In the case of someone who has had moderate sun exposure from a young age, the effect of all those UV rays means that in a couple of decades' time, their skin might look around 10 or 15 years older than it really is.

Youth in a jar

When wrinkles strike, many people begin to wage war against them. In fact, last year in the US alone, $850 million were spent on anti-ageing products. And it's not just the vanity of the developed world, either. In

Below: Most face creams don't reach the lower layers of your skin, shown here in pink, where dehydrated and shrinking fibres of collagen and elastin cause fine lines and wrinkles.

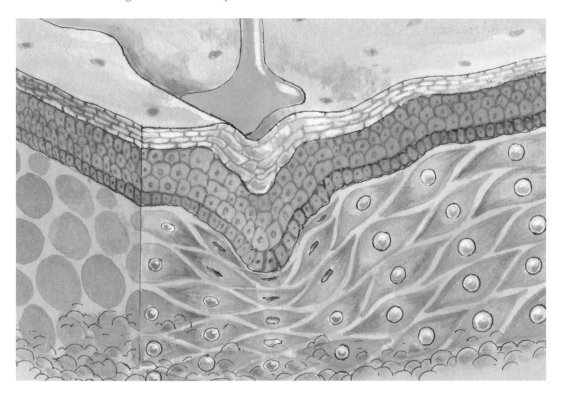

Right: A special camera with a UV light reveals sun damage, which can't be seen by the naked eye.

developing countries such as India, sales of anti-ageing creams are increasing by up to 40 per cent a year. The global beauty industry is on to a winner, but as people everywhere faithfully splash out on expensive pots of creams and lotions, what can science tell us about their effectiveness? To begin with, manufacturers harness science to lure us into buying their products. We know ageing is a biological process, so we seek out a scientifically proven course of treatment for it. All manner of pseudo-scientific words are liberally applied to anti-ageing products, each one, it seems, hiking the price up further. Take our test below to find out just how easily the beauty industry could tip you into making a purchase.

Applying science to beauty

Imagine that the following statements are on the label of an anti-ageing cream or lotion. Tick the ones that would suggest to you that the product in question had been proven to work:

a 'Contains active natural extracts that were shown to reduce fine lines and wrinkles in dermatological tests'

b 'With retinol – scientifically proven to eliminate wrinkles'

c 'With bio-vitamins to combat free radicals and regenerate and rejuvenate your skin'

d 'Contains patented proteins designed to moisturize and regenerate the skin'

e 'With a combination of anti-oxidants and fruit acids to detoxify your skin and reduce the signs of ageing'

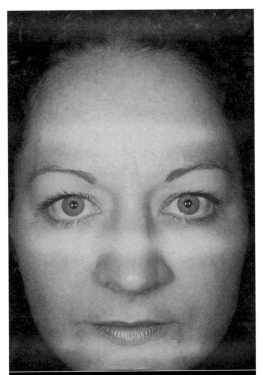
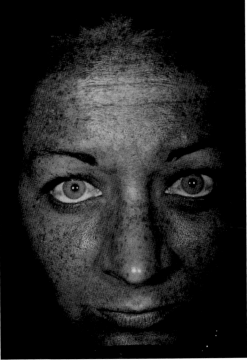

If you ticked any or all of the above statements, you might be parting with your money too readily. The fact is that while cosmetics companies must test their products before putting them on sale, they are not put through the kind of rigorous clinical tests that medicines are subjected to. In fact, research has shown that beauty manufacturers spend just 2 to 3 per cent of their profits on research and development, while most pharmaceutical companies spend around 15 per cent. Compare that with the 20 to 25 per cent it's estimated most cosmetics firms spend on marketing and promotion. Manufacturers know that science sells these kind of products but it's well worth analyzing advertising claims carefully for pseudo-science. Consider the following facts:

● Vague terms like 'active natural extracts', 'proteins' or 'bio-vitamins' don't count for much at all. All ingredients – by their very nature – are active, otherwise there would be no point in including them in a product. 'Natural' doesn't necessarily mean it's going to be gentler – in fact, face creams advertising lots of natural ingredients may even contain higher than average amounts of chemical preservatives to halt the growth of bacteria in them. Proteins and vitamins may well be included in face creams, but from a biological point of view they have no effect. You need to ingest proteins and vitamins for them to work: they cannot be absorbed by your skin, or by your nails or hair for that matter. These substances will only penetrate to the outer layers of your skin – while the effects of ageing might be seen there, they're actually taking place deep within your skin in the dermis layer.

● Nearly ten years ago, dermatologists found that a treatment for acne – a derivative of vitamin A called retinoic acid – seemed to be having an interesting side effect on patients: it was reducing wrinkles and producing younger-looking skin. After a huge battery of expensive clinical trials, retinoic acid was finally approved by the US Food and Drug Administration as a clinically effective means of reducing wrinkles and signs of premature ageing. Also known as Retin-A, Renova or Retinova, the cream must be used for a long period of time before any results are seen. However, it is available by prescription only as it can lead to serious side effects including skin redness, irritation, extreme dryness and excessive sensitivity to sunlight. For these reasons, cosmetics firms are banned from including it in over-the-counter face creams. Instead, they use a substance called retinol, a much less aggressive version of vitamin A, which most dermatologists agree is unlikely to have any significant anti-ageing effects.

● Just because a cosmetic product is more expensive, doesn't mean that it's more likely to work: in fact, you're probably just paying for more luxurious packaging or because a well-known brand name can get away with charging over the odds.

● If you do see positive effects after using an anti-ageing product, don't be fooled. The chances are these are mostly down to the moisturizing effect of slathering on a face cream. The fact is that almost all moisturizers work in exactly the same way, whether you splash out on a celebrity-endorsed 'wonder cream' or buy an inexpensive basic moisturizing product. They leave a thin layer of oil on the skin's surface that makes it feel and appear more supple and soft. That will also make fine lines appear reduced, as they'll be more hydrated and so plumped up. If you're not convinced, do a test of your own: try a brand-name face cream for a month, then swap to an economy version such as aqueous cream, which is available extremely cheaply from most pharmacies. While the packaging and fragrance of the latter might not give you that pampered feel, it's probably working in an almost identical way.

• Remember that no face cream you buy from the beauty counter is physically able to rejuvenate or regenerate the structure of your skin. If you can afford to buy expensive face creams and you fancy using a luxury product, then go ahead, but don't be tricked into thinking that it's going to make you wake up looking twenty years younger. Almost all dermatologists agree that there are two simple ways to slow down the signs of ageing: give up smoking and protect yourself from the sun's UV rays. Start applying a good-quality sun protection cream to your face every day, whether or not you live in a hot country. Some of the sun's rays (UVA) can even penetrate glass, so the odd bit of cloud isn't going to stop them. Don't rely on sun protection factors included in moisturizers or make-up, as you won't apply enough of the product to give your skin adequate UV protection. Instead, invest in an oil-free face sun protection cream with an SPF of at least 15 and use it every day. When it comes to being outdoors during the summer months or going on a hot holiday, refer to our advice in the section called 'Here comes the sun' in Chapter 4 (see pages 83–5).

• Finally, while you can try to halt signs of ageing by protecting your skin from harmful UV rays and the effects of smoking, do bear in mind that with time, your skin will inevitably lose its elasticity and develop wrinkles. Of course, you can opt for chemical injections and treatments or even plastic surgery to make yourself look younger. But laughter lines and wrinkles are reflections of your character, an expression of the years you've been through and the experiences you've gained. If you can learn to embrace them as the road map of your life so far, you're likely to improve your overall sense of self-esteem and wellbeing.

When whiffs strike

Just when you thought there couldn't possibly be another personal grooming issue your skin could throw at you, dig a little deeper and you'll hit the sweat glands. You've got around four million of these spread out across your body. The main purpose of perspiring is to keep your body temperature regulated. If you get too hot, the release of sweat means your skin will be cooled as the moisture evaporates. While you may think of sweating as nothing more than a minor nuisance, it's actually an intricate and clever system. Have a peek at your back in the mirror – in each square centimetre of skin, you'll have an incredible 60 sweat glands, while on the palms of your hands and soles of your feet, there'll be an amazing 600 glands in each square centimetre of skin.

It's not the sweat itself that causes the unpleasant whiff of body odour, but those usually harmless bacteria which, as we saw earlier, can get into blocked pores, wreaking all sorts of pimply havoc. Sweat is the perfect fertilizer for them to breed in, and as they reproduce, they produce rather smelly, pungent fatty acids. While most people taking things at a fairly sedate pace in a cool environment probably only produce around half a litre (1 pint) of sweat each day, those sweat glands can sometimes get bigger ideas. In fact, they've got the potential to produce up to 12 litres (21 pints) of sweat in just 24 hours. Of course, the more sweat, the more bacteria there are enjoying the moist, warm environment, so the greater the chance you'll have bad body odour. If you're concerned about sweating or body odour, or you've noticed you seem to sweat more than other people, follow our top tips below.

Top tips for coping with sweating

- **Wash regularly.** This will ensure that sweat and the bacteria that breed in it are kept at bay.

- **Don't wear clothes more than once without washing them.** Sweat goes stale in clothing and will smell even worse on the second day. Wash clothes at a hot temperature, especially items such as tops, shirts, underwear and socks that come into direct contact with your sweaty areas.

- **Always use anti-perspirant deodorants.** If you feel the one you're using isn't doing its job, check out some other products. Each one has different ingredients (check the label) and some brands might work better for you than others.

- **Shave your armpits.** The bacteria that grow in sweat and make those nasty whiffs can get an even better foothold if there's hair for them to hang on to.

- **Wear more natural fibres.** Synthetic materials make it harder for your skin to breathe, so it will sweat more quickly.

- **Wear leather shoes.** If smelly feet are a problem, pick leather shoes and make sure they've got a leather lining, not a plastic one. If you tend to wear trainers all the time, they won't be helping the problem – they're made entirely of synthetic material, which means your feet can't 'breathe' at all. So it's best to avoid wearing them for long periods of time.

- **Try a specific treatment.** If you've tried a multitude of deodorants and still feel that your body odour is a problem, consider buying an over-the-counter treatment called chlorhexidine 0.05% solution. This won't curb the sweating itself, but it will help to keep the bacteria at bay, so reducing your odour.

- **Ask your pharmacist's advice.** If the problem is more a case of excessive sweating rather than body odour, ask your pharmacist for 20 per cent aluminium chloride, which you can apply to your armpits when you go to bed. It blocks up the sweat glands to keep excessive wetness at bay, but make sure you read the instructions carefully – if it's used incorrectly it can irritate your skin and stain clothes.

- **Consult your doctor.** If you've tried all of the above tips and you're still finding you have a problem, it's worth visiting your doctor. Excessive sweating can be a symptom of some medical conditions. Once you get the all-clear, your doctor can advise you on a number of other options including botox injections into the sweat glands or even a couple of types of surgery, if your problem is more severe.

Mane misery

While women might get in a frenzy at how fast the crows' feet, fine lines and wrinkles are appearing on their faces, men tend to look over and above all that – at their receding hairlines. The simple fact is that in our culture, thick, lustrous hair is usually associated with youth, vitality and attractiveness, and baldness with ageing, illness and even immorality. Can you name more than a handful of very successful bald film stars or even one bald Western political leader? So it's no surprise that men don't tend to welcome hair loss with open arms.

Human hair is made of keratin, a strong protein that also forms the outer layer of your skin and nails. As you'll see in the illustration below, each hair root lies under the surface of the skin in a protective pit called the follicle. On average, you've probably got around 100,000 hairs sprouting from these follicles across your scalp (if that sounds like a lot, bear in mind that there are 5 million hair follicles all over your body, but the vast majority of these just produce tiny fuzz-like hairs that are hardly noticeable).

Astonishingly, each of the hairs on your head survives for two to six years, growing about 1 cm (³⁄₈ inch) each month. After this phase, the hair stops growing altogether for about five to six weeks; then it becomes detached from the follicle and either falls out or is pushed out by a new hair, which takes its place to begin a new growth/rest cycle. At any moment, about 85 per cent of the hair

Below: In some men, high levels of the hormone DHT (seen here in yellow) circulate in the blood, causing hair follicles in the scalp to shrink over time and produce much weaker hairs that eventually fall out.

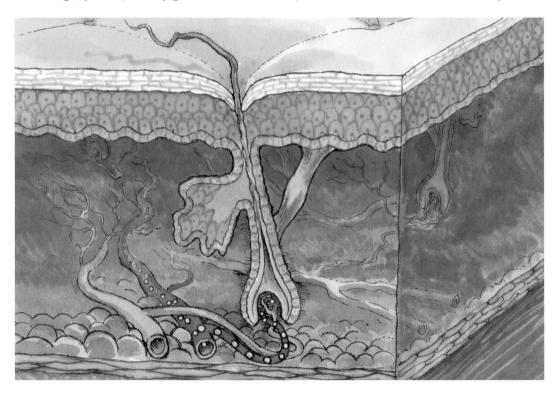

follicles on your head are in the growth phase and the remainder are resting. Each hair goes through the growth/rest cycle completely independently of its neighbours, so the total number of hairs is usually pretty constant with an average of 50 to 100 falling out each day.

Male pattern hair loss (known as androgenetic alopecia) is by far the most common form of baldness. About 15 per cent of men have obviously begun to lose their hair by the time they reach 30 and moderate hair loss affects about half of all men aged 45 or over. It usually takes the form of a receded hair line at the front of the head and a bald area at the crown and mid-scalp. Mysteriously, the hair at the sides of the head is almost always unaffected. So what triggers this loss of hair? Basically, it's all about androgens – the male sex hormones. Scientists believe that a combination of androgens and a genetic predisposition to androgen-sensitivity mark you out for baldness to some degree. The culprit androgen is dihydrotestosterone (DHT), which is converted from testosterone by an enzyme, 5-alpha reductase. It's thought that excess levels of DHT cause a shortening of the growth phase and a gradual reduction of follicle size in some areas of the scalp. Over time, more hair follicles find themselves in a longer resting stage and begin to shrink across each new growth phase, producing hairs that become finer and less pigmented until eventually they die altogether.

Keep your hair on

The vast number of alleged 'miracle cures' for baldness gives a hint of how some men will try anything and everything to keep their hair, from useless expensive potions to flimsy hairpieces and supposedly ground-breaking procedures such as hair transplantation. The original transplant technique, developed in the 1980s, involved moving areas of healthy hair follicles from the back of the head to the front and top. But this procedure generally produced a sprouting, doll-like hair line and a clumpy and unconvincing top area. Today, things have moved on somewhat, with more fine-grained transplanting techniques in use, but there are now more promising drug treatments on the market.

There are two anti-baldness drugs currently approved by the US Food and Drug Administration as being clinically effective, although don't expect miracles. The first on the market was a drug called minoxidil (marketed as Regaine). Originally a blood pressure medication, it's unclear how it works in cases of hair loss, but it's now widely available over the counter as a lotion that is applied to the scalp. It may encourage your hair to remain in its growth phase for longer. The hairs that do regrow are often downy and fine and the benefits gradually reverse if you stop using the product.

More recently, scientists noted that people with a rare deficiency of the 5-alpha reductase enzyme rarely went bald. This encouraged the pharmaceutical giants to set their sights on finding ways of inhibiting DHT action (see above) – cue a drug called finasteride (marketed in the UK as Propecia). Tests on this drug show that four out of five men maintain or increase their amount of hair, with noticeable benefits starting at around six months after starting a course of finasteride. As with minoxidil, the effects gradually fade off if you stop taking the tablets. A few patients have reported some unwanted sexual side effects (including decreased libido, reduced semen volume and slight loss of erection), which disappear on stopping the drug.

Top ten tips for coping with hair loss

- **Don't buy dubious lotions.** And don't spend your hard-earned cash on supplements advertised in magazines or on the Internet – they won't work.

- **Don't wash or brush your hair less.** It won't make any difference to your hair falling out, and if it's attractiveness to others that you're concerned about, there's nothing like poor hygiene or lack of grooming to put someone off.

- **Don't cover up.** Hiding your thinning hair under a baseball cap is hardly a lifelong fashion option and will just serve to highlight how uncomfortable you feel about your hair loss.

- **Don't grow a beard.** Trying to compensate for the diminishing hair on your head by nurturing your facial hair will make your face look heavy and add years to it.

- **Don't cultivate a comb-over to cover up thinning patches.** Not only is this a global fashion no-no, the bottom line is you're not going to kid anyone.

- **Consider shaving your head.** It's a bold fashion statement that reflects confidence and a positive choice. If this is not the look for you, at least consider having your remaining hair cut short to counter the thinner or bald patches.

- **Try an approved treatment.** Look for minoxidil (available over the counter) or finasteride (available on prescription from a doctor). Don't get your hopes up too much, but stick with the treatment for at least six months and you will hopefully see a slight improvement.

- **Share your worries with your partner or friends.** If you feel embarrassed about it, try to overcome your concerns by remembering that hair loss is extremely common in men. By bringing the issue out into the open, you'll hopefully lessen some of your concerns and get reassurance and support.

- **Do try to limit your anxiety.** It's all too easy for concerns to grow into obsessions. Remember, there's not a huge amount you can do to stop the process but uncontrolled anxiety about it could end up affecting your health. If you find yourself checking how many hairs have fallen out on to your pillow each morning, or if you're constantly looking in the mirror at your hairline, things could be starting to get out of hand. Consider contacting a local hair-loss support group or talk to your doctor about the situation.

- **Concentrate on the rest of your body.** There are many ways you can improve your appearance and attractiveness: keep your face, hands and nails clean and groomed, update your wardrobe as often as you can and, most importantly of all, exercise regularly to improve your overall fitness and physique. The vast majority of women would much rather go out with a fit, toned, bald guy than an overweight hairy one.

While both these drugs aren't cures as such, they seem to offer the first truly effective treatment for male hair loss – and however small the positive effects are, men are prepared to pay: it's estimated that $400 million a year is spent on such medications. Until better results can be promised, researchers struggle on to find better treatments. In the next ten years, advances in genetic engineering may enable scientists to take a few healthy donor hair follicles from a patient, use them to cultivate a number of new hair cells and then surgically implant these where they're needed on the scalp. Until then, if your thinning hair is getting you down, take a look at our top tips (see opposite) to help boost your hair-esteem.

Body beautiful

It's human nature to compare ourselves with others as a way of trying to place ourselves in the complex tapestry of society. But as the age-old social divisions of class, wealth, education and religion have been progressively stripped away, a new means of judging ourselves has come to the fore over the past few decades. Our bodies, and in particular, their weight, shape and fitness, have become a sort of personal billboard for who we are, how happy we are and how well we're doing in life. Combine that with enormous media-fuelled pressure to conform to a certain look, add a big dose of cultural stigma should you fail to achieve that look and you have the perfect recipe for untold levels of insecurity, dissatisfaction and downright misery. Your body is at the very core of your identity – how you feel about it is not just a matter of vain, superficial concern, but one that, if left to fester, can impact hugely on your happiness, self-esteem and overall wellbeing.

If your mind is regularly filled with thoughts about what the scales said this morning, how you looked in the mirror in a particular pair of trousers or how a beautiful fashion model in a magazine made you feel, you are far from alone. A recent psychological survey of nearly 5000 people all over the world showed that 56 per cent of women and 43 per cent of men are unhappy with the way their body looks. Weight plays a huge part in their dissatisfaction: nearly 90 per cent of women who took the survey wanted to lose weight, with 15 per cent of women and 11 per cent of men admitting that they'd sacrifice more than five years of their life if they could be their goal weight. What's more, among smokers, a shocking 50 per cent of women and 30 per cent of men questioned said that one of the main reasons they chose to smoke cigarettes was to control their weight. While we all know that people suffering from eating disorders take extreme and dangerous measures to achieve what they perceive as the ideal body, what's surprising here is just how many 'normal' people seem more than willing to risk heart and lung disease, cancer or even death in their quest to achieve the ideal body.

To get an idea of just how desperately people want to alter their bodies to fit into our culture's extraordinarily narrow limits of beauty, you only have to look at the ever-growing numbers of people choosing to have cosmetic surgery. In 2002, 6.5 million Americans visited a plastic surgeon for purely aesthetic reasons. Of those, 1.6 million went under the knife, with the most popular procedures being nose re-shaping, liposuction, breast implants, eyelid surgery and facelifts. The remaining 4.9 million chose non-surgical procedures, such as botox injections to smooth wrinkles, chemical

Rate your body image wellbeing

1 How do you feel about undressing in a communal changing room, say in a clothing shop, gym or swimming pool?
I'd have no problem with it at all = 0 points
I'd be a bit embarrassed, but I'd just do it as quickly as possible = 1 point
I'd be very embarrassed and would try to conceal my body = 2 points
I wouldn't consider getting undressed in front of others = 3 points

Your score ☐

2 When it comes to sex, how do you feel about a partner seeing you naked?
I positively enjoy my partner seeing my whole body naked = 0 points
I'm embarrassed about my body at the start of a sexual relationship, but gradually I relax = 1 point
There are a few parts of my body that I try to conceal with bedding, clothing or by making sure we only have sex in certain positions = 2 points
I make sure we only have sex at night with the lights off = 3 points

Your score ☐

3 When you look at yourself in the mirror, how do you generally feel?
There are a few things about my body that I'd like to change or improve, but I generally feel OK about it = 0 points
There are a few things about my body that upset me occasionally when I look in the mirror = 1 point
There's one thing about my body in particular that upsets me every time I look in the mirror = 2 points
I try never to look at myself in the mirror = 3 points

Your score ☐

4 If you could be more physically attractive, how would it change your life?
I'd probably be a bit more confident, but it wouldn't change much else about my life = 0 points
I'd be far happier = 1 point
I'd be more successful and popular = 2 points
My partner or a potential partner would like me more = 3 points

Your score ☐

5 **Think about the thing or things you dislike most about your body. How do they make you feel?**
The feature I'm concerned about runs in my family so I know there's not that much I can do about it = 0 points
I should try to improve what I don't like through diet or exercise = 1 point
I don't try nearly hard enough to improve myself = 2 points
There's no point trying to improve myself as I know I could never achieve the body I really want = 3 points

Your score ☐

6 **Think back to last week. How often did thinking about or looking at your body make you feel concerned, anxious or insecure?**
Never = 0 points
Once or twice = 1 point
Every day = 2 points
Several times every day = 3 points

Your score ☐

Now add up your scores and enter your total ☐

What your score means:
0 to 7 = You have a very healthy body image. Remember, it's normal to be concerned with how your body looks and you should harness this to make sure you keep fit and healthy. If your feelings about your body ever get worse or change depending on your mood or after a particular negative experience, take the test again to ensure you're not slipping into bad body image habits.

8 to 12 = Your score suggests that body image concerns could be affecting your life and wellbeing. Follow our top tips on page 108 to make sure your feelings don't get out of control. There are plenty of ways you can learn to feel better about your body. If you don't feel any differently after trying out a few of these, consider speaking to your doctor or a counsellor about the situation.

13 to 18 = The way you feel about your body seems to be significantly impacting on how you live your life and feel about yourself. These negative thoughts can distort the way you perceive your body, triggering even more insecurity, anxiety and critical thinking. It would be a good idea to ask your doctor about some counselling to help you improve your feelings about your body.

Top tips for feeling good about your body

- **Make a list of all the positive things you feel you've achieved in the past (but do not include any that relate to your appearance).** The list might include job successes, achieving goals in your career, travelling to places you always wanted to go or supporting family and friends through difficult times. Now make a second list of your future goals in the same categories. When concerns about your body creep into your mind, read both lists again and try to focus your mind on the positive ways you judge yourself in life.

- **Learn to appreciate the bits you don't like.** Pick the part of your body you dislike the most. Now make a list of all the physical functions that body part enables you to do. How would your life be affected if you didn't have it at all? In other words, try to nurture an appreciation of how miraculous your body really is – that way you'll gradually build up levels of satisfaction.

- **Replace negative thoughts about your body with positive actions.** When you get into a mental rut about how you look, do something you know will lift your mood such as exercising or speaking to a supportive friend. Don't let bad thoughts breed even worse ones.

- **Treat your body with respect.** Eat healthily, exercise regularly and give your body a treat whenever you can – that could be a long, soothing bath, a new body moisturizing cream or a relaxing massage.

- **Accentuate the positive.** Next time you're shopping for clothes, try to choose items that enhance or show off the bits of your body you feel positively about. If you can work up even a little bit of pride for one part of your body, it will improve how you feel about the rest.

- **Ban yourself from buying fashion magazines.** If you've got body image concerns, constantly looking at ultra-skinny or unusually beautiful fashion models and celebrities is only going to make you feel far worse. Remember that almost all photographs in magazines get air-brushed to improve the way models and stars look, so you're probably mentally beating yourself up over nothing more than a computer-enhanced image. Even in magazines that claim they don't condone the use of overly thin models, you'll find any number of comments on celebrity weight loss or gain, and bodies and figures 'to die for'. If you want to feel better about yourself, stop reading them.

- **Eliminate negativity not just in yourself, but in others too.** If your friends or acquaintances make snipes about the way you look or your partner criticizes your body, you seriously need to rethink why these people are in your life. Surround yourself with people who respect you for who you are and find a partner who positively enjoys your body. Remember you need to think, feel and experience positivity as much as you can to help you get over body image concerns.

- **Get help and support.** If you've tried all of the above for a good few weeks and you find your mind is still filled with negative thoughts about your body, it's probably worth seeing your doctor or a counsellor to try and tackle the problem. By actively choosing to deal with your body image issues, you'll be well on the way to improving your confidence, self-worth and overall wellbeing.

Below: Taking the time to respect and enjoy your body will have positive benefits for your wellbeing.

peels and microdermabrasion, to improve skin texture. While a quick nip and tuck might be the easiest (albeit not the cheapest) way to eliminate something you really hate about your body once and for all, it won't alter the underlying belief that to be happy and successful, you need to look a certain way. Take our body image test on pages 106–7 to find out how much your own feelings about your body might be affecting your overall health and wellbeing.

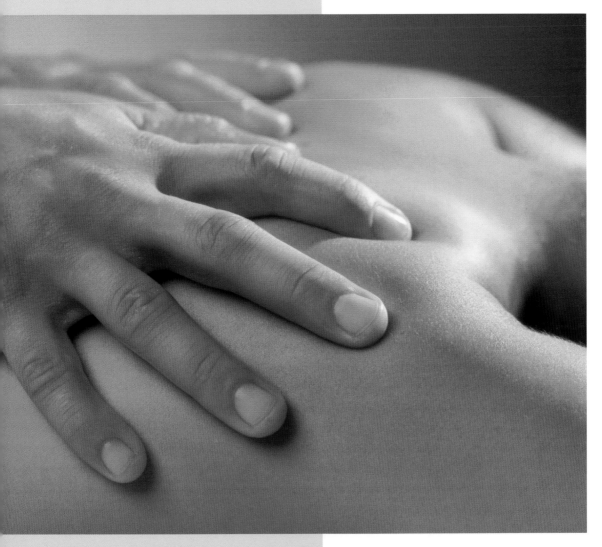

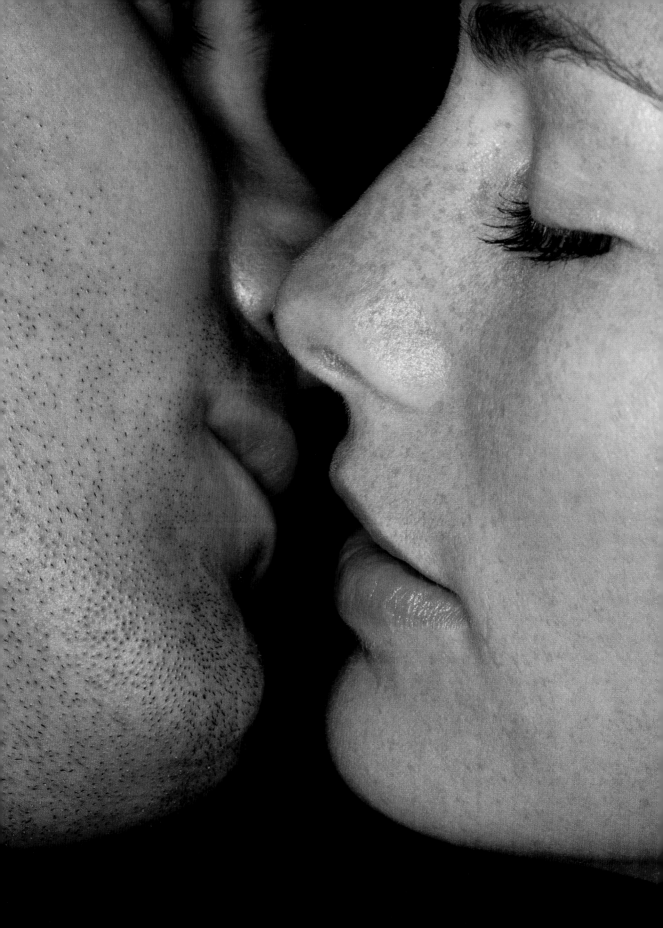

6

Love, Sex & Making Babies

Caring about your appearance reflects the most vital of all our instincts: the drive to reproduce. The animal urge to attract the ideal mate for a bit of gene-sharing influences our behaviour in relationships far more than we realize. But being rather more complex than basic beasts, our biological quest for offspring comes packaged in a deeply elaborate emotional and physical concoction of attraction, romance, love and passion. Such is the magical power of affairs of the heart that most of us don't stop to consider the physiology and psychology behind them. In this chapter, we'll reveal the science of why you're attracted to some people and not others, what happens inside your body and brain when you fall for someone and how your body's reaction to sex can tip you head over heels into love, whether you like it or not!

As we saw earlier, the human body evolved a reward response to eating because it was so important for our species' survival – in much the same way, reproduction also evolved to be highly pleasurable. You even have a hormonal drive to seek sexual pleasure out, just in case it should slip your mind. And that drive works exceptionally well – during the course of today alone, 100 million acts of sexual intercourse will take place around the world.

While we tend to think of pleasure first and foremost when it comes to sex, there also comes a time in most people's lives when sex means babies. We'll uncover what's going on inside your body when you're 'trying for a baby' and what you can do to optimize your fertility. There's also a guide to what causes fertility problems and we'll explain the various infertility treatments on offer.

Who do you fancy?

You're looking at someone who's drop-dead gorgeous. What exactly is it about them that's so attractive to you? You'd probably put it down to their sexy body, stylish looks, interesting face or even their personality. The chances are that the very last thing you're likely to rate as attractive is someone's genetic make-up, but in the science of attraction, genes matter. While you might think choosing your ideal partner is all about making conscious decisions, we're all hugely controlled by our unconscious drive to further our genes by reproducing. And that means getting together with someone who carries the kind of genes that'll ensure your kids go on to be healthy, attractive and therefore have children of their own.

The first adults you ever saw were most probably your parents. They were your models of an adult male and female and in the most simple terms, they imprinted on your mind the basic image of what sort of person you'd look to pair with in later life. Studies have shown that if a baby duck happens to get raised with a family of geese, it will try to mate with a goose when it reaches maturity. Of course, you didn't need to take a glance at your mother or father to know that you're not meant to mate with another species, but a number of subtle messages about your type of ideal partner probably did become etched into your unconscious mind as you grew up.

Firstly, your physical appearance reflects what type of genes you've got, so the way you and your family look gives you some important clues about your individual genetic make-up. It stands to reason then that in the quest to further your genes you might be more attracted to a partner who resembles you physically – it would mean an even

greater chance that your genes would get passed on in the DNA-shuffling process that takes place during sexual reproduction. As part of BBC3's *Body Hits* series, we put this theory to the test. John was a guinea-pig for a team of researchers from St Andrews University in Scotland. He had been told that the scientists would simply be looking at what sort of female faces he found attractive, but that wasn't strictly the truth. They had obtained a photograph of John's face and had digitally manipulated the image so that some of his facial features were added into a number of photographs of female faces. When it came to the test, John was shown a series of pairs of female faces. In each pair, one face secretly contained some of his own facial features, albeit in feminized form. Would he be more attracted to the faces that shared his own characteristics? Amazingly, the results showed that 70 per cent of the time, he was rating the female faces that more closely resembled his own as the most attractive, without even realizing why.

While lookalike faces might reflect potential partners who share some of the same genes, choosing a partner who's too similar could have disastrous consequences. Inbreeding means there's a far greater chance that genes for rare disorders will get passed on to new generations. The universal taboo of incest shows just how strongly cultures try to prevent inbreeding from happening. Besides which, choosing a partner who's quite different has some major biological bonuses.

Opposites attract

When it comes to thinking about the attractiveness of a potential partner, we can be pretty sure that their immune system doesn't cross your mind – your conscious mind, that is. Surprisingly enough, the genes that define what type of immune system you have are the most varied of all in the human genotype, which means there are millions of unique types. What's more, scientists have discovered that your immune system and the way you smell are closely linked.

In an intriguing study, Swiss researchers asked a group of men to wear a cotton T-shirt in bed every night for several nights. The men were asked not to wear cologne, deodorant or even to wash before wearing the T-shirts. Then a group of women was asked to have a good sniff of the T-shirts and rate how attractive each one smelled. Interestingly, they each preferred the smell of the man whose immune system was most different from their own. If you think about it, that makes good

sense. Each type of immune system confers protection against a different selection of bugs and infections, so by choosing a partner with an immune system that varies greatly from your own, you're unconsciously ensuring that any children you have with that partner end up with even better immune protection than your own.

But just as inbreeding is the extreme end of choosing a partner with too many similarities, so by going for a partner with too many different characteristics, you end up with what's known as outbreeding – and mating with other species certainly isn't your best option for having healthy kids!

Below: Looks attract us, but unconsciously we seek out similar genes and a good immune system.

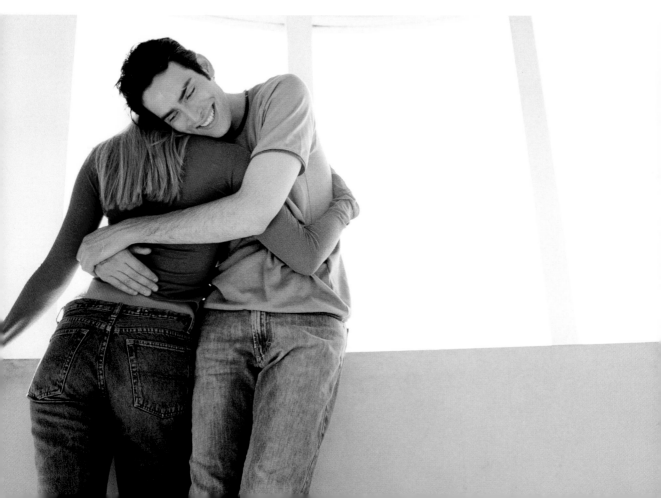

Instead, your biology drives you to find a partner who's the perfect compromise between sameness and difference and you unconsciously try to strike that balance in all sorts of physical and behavioural characteristics, not just when it comes to being attracted to certain faces or smells.

Weak at the knees

You might not be able to put your finger on what it is about a person that triggers it, but you'll certainly know when it happens. When you meet someone you're attracted to a chemical firework display kicks off inside your mind and body, and its effects are responsible for the delicious sensations that make up that first stage of love – attraction and lust. Information about your love object's looks, smell and what they're saying and doing gets conveyed through your eyes, ears and nose to your brain. It heads straight to your amygdala, the tiny almond-shaped object that processes all your emotions.

As you'll see in the illustration below, the amygdala triggers a cascade of chemicals including the hormones adrenaline and noradrenaline, which surge right through the body. Working together, they'll make your heart pound up to three times faster than normal and divert your blood supplies away from areas that aren't top priority, such as your stomach (that's why you'll experience the feeling of butterflies there). Instead, the blood is hastily sent to your cheeks, providing a sexy flush – a handy marker of sexual

Below: The amygdala (seen here in green) triggers a cascade of adrenaline and noradrenaline that excites your brain when you're attracted to someone. Meanwhile, a flood of dopamine gives you a high.

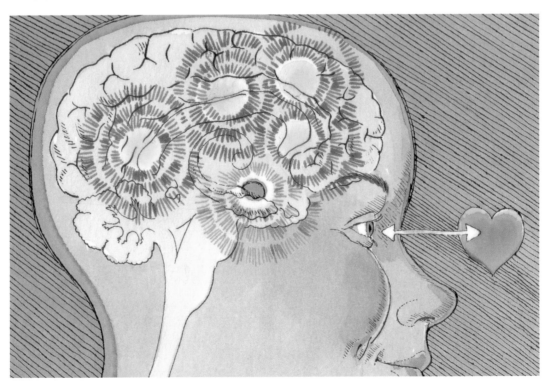

arousal for your potential partner – and of course, directly to your genitals: let's not forget, after all, that while you might be thinking of romance and love, your body's gearing up for sex and reproduction.

It's not just your body that's firing on all cylinders either: deep inside your brain, as the illustration opposite also shows, there are major stirrings too. As we saw earlier (see page 56), dopamine is the natural brain chemical that is so intrinsically linked to pleasure (and, indeed, is the means by which many drugs produce their chemical highs). It gets released in four key areas of your brain when you're with someone you're falling for. Interestingly, those are the same parts of the brain that pump up dopamine levels if you take cocaine. No wonder then that falling in love produces a natural high, which makes you feel energized, excited and full of joy.

Sex meets love

While of course it's possible to have sex with someone without falling madly in love with them, if you have enough sex with the same person, there's a good chance you'll discover your body's got a few tricks up its sleeve to bond you to that partner. Affectionate touching and stroking, cuddling and, most of all, orgasm all produce surges of a feel-good hormone called oxytocin. Animal studies have shown that oxytocin helps partners form close emotional pair-bonds. One project looked at prairie voles – animals that usually form close monogamous bonds for many years. The study compared two groups of voles: one with normal brains and the other whose special brain receptors for oxytocin were not working properly. In the second group, the animals simply didn't pair off at all and showed no attachment to each other.

In theory the more sex you have with your partner, the deeper your emotional bond becomes as a result of that regular oxytocin release. But differences between men's and women's bodies might get in the way – some scientists think that when oxytocin combines with the female hormone, oestrogen, it can make a woman feel very cuddly and chatty after sex, but when it combines with the male hormone testosterone, it can trigger an instant post-orgasmic urge to sleep. It seems our bodies haven't yet mastered post-coital harmony between the sexes!

Head over heels

Being in love is a euphoric experience that can make people do wild, irrational things, feel joyous and find themselves head over heels. That chemical cocktail inside your brain and body is extremely powerful, acting like a natural drug to bring about all the wonderful physical and emotional sensations of being in love. That's worth bearing in mind if you've ever wondered why the end of a relationship has made you feel so bad – especially if it was your partner rather than you who chose to end the relationship.

Before you jump to the conclusion that rejection is just rather embarrassing, new research has shown that it causes very real pain deep inside your brain. A team at the University of California in Los Angeles asked a group of subjects to play a computer game while they lay inside an MRI brain-scanner. They were told that the other players in the virtual game were being controlled by unseen researchers. The game involved simple ball-catching between the players, but after a few minutes of being included in the computer-generated gang, the subject was unceremoniously ignored and didn't get to throw the ball again. As you can imagine, the experience probably sparked a few distressing childhood playground memories for most of the subjects, but the MRI data showed some more intriguing results. Being snubbed in the game triggered brain activity in a region called the anterior cingulate cortex, which is known to be a major player in the brain's response to physical pain. Being rejected by a partner would be a much greater emotional snub than being left out in a ball-game, so the pain response is likely to be far greater.

Just as drug addicts start to feel withdrawal symptoms if they haven't had a fix for a while, the sudden withdrawal of love also has marked effects on the brain's chemical balance. It takes a while for your brain and body to adapt to the lack of that delicious chemical love cocktail that it's become accustomed to. You might feel cravings for that love 'high', which combined with the pain of rejection can leave you feeling very low emotionally, something which most people experience at the end of an important relationship. With time, the love withdrawal symptoms will fade, but in the interim, the experience can be devastating.

The crazy stage

It seems that whether you're in love or lovesick, the chemical cocktail working inside your brain and body has the power to tip you over the edge into very irrational, uncontrolled behaviour. That craziness of love has inspired thousands of writers, artists and musicians across the ages. But rather than just being a strange by-product of our ability to form a bond with a partner, some experts believe there's a good reason for crazy love.

In a US research study, 5000 people from 37 different cultures around the world were interviewed about love and relationships.

Intriguingly, the results showed that most people experienced the heady, out-of-control sensations of being in love for between just 18 to 30 months at the start of a relationship. After that, relationships either broke up or entered a more gentle phase of long-term attachment. Evolutionary psychologists claim that's because the first delicious stage of love is all about reproducing – for our ancient ancestors, 18 to 30 months would have been just long enough for a pair to meet, mate and get a child on two feet, after which they could then move on and have another go with a new partner, ensuring that their genes got spread as widely as possible. The theory goes that unless our ancestors had been absorbed in the craziness of love, they might not have wanted to undertake the chore of having kids in the first place. While it's not the most romantic explanation, perhaps the pleasure of being in love – in much the same way as our reward response to eating or sex – truly is one of evolution's cunning tricks to ensure our survival.

When two becomes three

When your 'wild oats' are all sown and you've found a partner you want to settle down with, new priorities appear on the horizon and they often include the patter of tiny feet. If you make it through the heady first stage of being in love, your brain produces a new chemical mix as you head into long-term attachment. It releases endorphins – the pain-relieving, calming chemicals that, as we saw in Chapter 3, are produced when you exercise (see page 58). In this case, it is thought that they help to smooth over the everyday issues and hiccups of being in a long-term

Right: Your lifestyle choices can make a big difference to your chances of having a baby.

relationship – and for those couples hoping to be parents, a bit of pain-relieving may go a long way!

Getting pregnant is much harder than most people think. Of the 100 million acts of sexual intercourse taking place around the world today, only 910,000 will result in conceptions. That means that over 99 million couples will fail to get pregnant. Of course, many of those are actively trying to prevent a pregnancy by using contraception, but even when coils, caps and condoms aren't involved, achieving a pregnancy can be a difficult business.

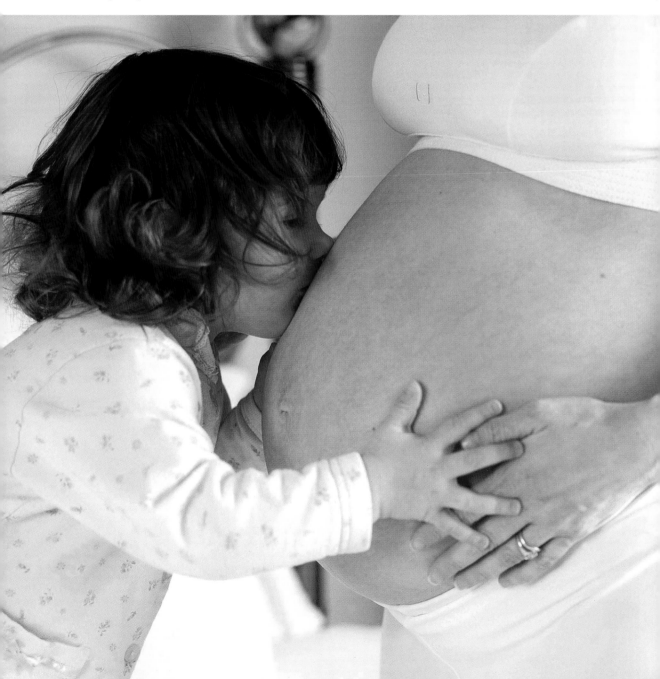

Rate lifestyle effects on your fertility

Part 1: For women only

1 What is your age?
Under 25 = 0 points
25 to 35 = 1 point
35 to 45 = 3 points
Over 45 = 4 points

Your score ☐

2 Look back to Chapter 2 (see page 34) to find out how to work out your body mass index (BMI). What is it?
19 or below = 4 points
20 to 25 = 0 points
25 or above = 3 points

Your score ☐

3 Are you a smoker?
No, I've never smoked = 0 points
No, I gave up recently = 1 point
Yes, I smoke but I've cut down = 2 points
Yes, I smoke regularly = 3 points

Your score ☐

4 How often do you drink coffee or caffeinated soft drinks?
Never = 0 points
Probably a couple of times a week = 1 point
Once a day = 2 points
Several times a day = 3 points

Your score ☐

5 How often do you drink alcohol?
Never or fewer than 5 units a week = 0 points
Two to three units of alcohol a day (see page 22 for calculating units) = 1 point
21+ units of alcohol a week = 2 points

Your score ☐

6 Do you ever take drugs, such as cannabis or cocaine and if so, how often?
I don't take drugs = 0 points
I take cannabis, cocaine or other drugs very occasionally = 2 points
I take cannabis, cocaine or other drugs regularly = 4 points

Your score ☐

7 After you've had sex, what are you most likely to do?
Sleep or rest for 15 minutes or more = 0 points
Lie down for a few minutes and have a cuddle with your partner = 1 point
Get up and go to the bathroom, then return to bed = 2 points
Get up and get on with your day = 3 points

Your score ☐

8 Which of the following statements about stress applies to you?
I rarely feel stressed = 0 points
My job, family or relationship can occasionally be stressful = 1 point
I experience stress at home and/or work on a regular basis = 2 points
I regularly experience symptoms of stress, such as high blood pressure, sleeplessness and anxiety = 3 points

Your score ☐

Your total score for part 1 ☐

Part 2: For men only

1 What kind of underwear do you wear most regularly?
Boxer shorts = 0 points
Y-fronts = 3 points
Tight briefs = 4 points
Your score ☐

2 What type of trousers do you wear most regularly?
Loose casual style = 0 points
Suit trousers = 1 point
Tight jeans = 2 points
Your score ☐

3 Do you take a bath or a shower most regularly?
Always a shower = 0 points
A mixture of showers and baths = 2 points
Always a bath = 3 points
Your score ☐

4 Which of the following statements best describes your average working day?
I spend most of my day on my feet
= 0 points
I spend most of my day sitting down
= 2 points
Your score ☐

5 Are you a smoker?
No, I've never smoked = 0 points
No, I gave up recently = 1 point
Yes, I smoke but I've cut down = 2 points
Yes, I smoke regularly = 3 points
Your score ☐

6 How often do you drink alcohol?
Never or fewer than eight units a week
= 0 points
No more than 28 units a week (see page 22 for calculating units) = 1 point
28+ units of alcohol a week = 2 points
Your score ☐

7 Do you take drugs, such as cannabis or cocaine and if so, how often?
I never take drugs = 0 points
I take cannabis, cocaine or other drugs very occasionally = 2 points
I take cannabis, cocaine or other drugs regularly = 4 points
Your score ☐

8 Which of the following statements about stress applies to you?
I rarely feel stressed = 0 points
My job, family or relationship can occasionally be stressful = 1 point
I experience stress at home and/or work on a regular basis = 2 points
I regularly experience symptoms of stress, such as high blood pressure, sleeplessness and anxiety = 3 points
Your score ☐

Your total score for part 2 ☐

Part 3: For both of you – answer together

1 How long have you been actively trying to get pregnant?
We've only just started in the last few months = 0 points
We've been trying for under a year = 1 point
We've been trying for over a year = 2 points
We've been trying for over two years = 3 points

Your score ☐

2 How often do you have sex?
Every day = 0 points
A couple of times a week = 2 point
Every few weeks = 3 points
Once a month = 4 points

Your score ☐

3 In which position do you most regularly have sex?
Missionary = 0 points
From behind = 1 point
Woman on top = 2 points
Standing up = 3 points

Your score ☐

Your total score for part 3 ☐

Now add up the scores for each part in the boxes below to work out your combined total:

Part 1 (the woman's questions) ☐

Part 2 (the man's questions) ☐

Part 3 (the couple's questions) ☐

Grand total ☐

What your combined score means:
0 to 20 points = Your lifestyle choices shouldn't be impacting very much at all on your chances of getting pregnant. If you've been trying for around a year, keep going, but take a look at our top tips for improving your fertility (see pages 122–4) so that you stay on the right track. If you've been trying for two years and you've been having sex at least three or four times a week, speak to your doctor.

21 to 35 points = Some aspects of your lifestyle could be affecting your chances of getting pregnant. Follow our advice on pages 122–4 and try to alter some of your habits to optimize your chances of getting pregnant before you seek any medical help.

36 to 58 points = If you're serious about getting pregnant, you should try to change your lifestyle straight away or your chances of success could be substantially reduced. Take a look at our top tips for fertility on pages 122–4 for more details.

Let's consider the basic ingredients: a woman's eggs and a man's sperm, which happen to be the largest and smallest cells in the human body respectively. If you're a woman, you might be surprised to know that even by the fifth month of your foetal life in your mother's womb, you already had around 7 million eggs in your tiny ovaries. When you were born, more than half of those eggs had already died and from that moment on – although you might not have thought much about it for another 30 years or so – your biological clock began ticking. By puberty, only around 500,000 of your eggs were left, but with one dying off every 90 minutes or so, you'll only ever ovulate between 400 and 500 times during your fertile years.

For men, it's a very different story. You didn't start producing sperm until you hit puberty, but after that your testicles went haywire. On an average day, they should produce around 100 to 200 million sperm. Nevertheless, it's a complicated biological process and each sperm takes around three months to be completed. At any one time, you'll have sperm of all ages in your testicles – the youngest of which still have the whole three-month production period ahead of them.

While a sperm and egg get-together sounds simple enough, you also have to factor in that women only ovulate once a month (although recent findings suggest that some women may ovulate more than once in each cycle). Ovulation (when a mature egg is released from an ovary and can be fertilized) tends to happen in the middle of a woman's menstrual cycle, but that can vary hugely depending on many different biological factors. Just because you ovulate at a particular point in one cycle, it doesn't mean to say the next will be the same. Finally, bear in mind that while sperm can survive inside the woman's body for several days, a mature egg dies up to 24 hours after ovulation. That window for fertilization is really very small indeed.

On top of all that, how you choose to live your life can have a big impact on your chances of getting pregnant. For women, who carry their diminishing store of eggs with them from birth, lifestyle factors may have more of an effect as they'll be exposing all their eggs to them at any one time. For men, that three-month sperm production period means that lifestyle choices have a shorter-term effect. Over 80 million people worldwide are affected by infertility problems. Below we examine the various treatment options for people in that situation. However, if you're currently trying for a baby or planning to in the near future, it's well worth knowing how you can adapt your lifestyle to optimize your chances of getting pregnant. Take our specially designed three-part questionnaire on pages 118–20 to find out how your way of life might be affecting your chances.

Understanding infertility

Here's a capsule guide to the most common infertility causes and the treatments on offer, giving you a basic definition of the terms used and what they mean:

Infertility causes – apart from lifestyle factors that can inhibit fertility, there are several major causes of infertility. These include sperm dysfunctions, such as low counts or motility, ovulation disorders (as in the condition polycystic ovary syndrome or PCOS) or fallopian tube damage (where the tubes are blocked or damaged – as in the case of the sexually transmitted infection chlamydia which, as we will see in Chapter 7, can cause long-term pelvic inflammatory disease).

Top tips for improving your fertility

- **Don't leave it too late.** There's a good reason why women hear their biological clocks ticking. The peak age for fertility in women is during their twenties. But as many people now prefer having children later, it's worth bearing in mind that your chances of becoming pregnant in any one month decrease from 20 per cent in women over the age of 30 to 5 per cent in women over 40. While men's overall fertility doesn't decline in the same way, there is some evidence to suggest that sperm quality may be reduced after the age of 45.

- **Quit smoking.** While smoking is known to reduce men's sperm count and quality, its effects are far more significant on women's fertility. The toxic chemicals in cigarette smoke damage the tiny hairs or cilia that line a woman's fallopian tubes and help transport the egg from the ovary to the womb. Smoking may also affect the quality of a woman's eggs and increase the time it takes her to get pregnant – by up to 3.4 times longer than a non-smoker. Even if you've cut down the number of cigarettes you smoke, your fertility could still be affected. Studies have shown that smokers who reduce their daily number of cigarettes tend to inhale more deeply to get the same nicotine kick. If you want to get pregnant, you're going to have to stop anyway for the sake of your baby's health, so both of you should bite the bullet right now and give up (and don't forget that passive smoking counts too).

- **Cut down on toxins.** Alcohol, caffeine and illegal drugs all impact negatively on your fertility. In some studies it has been shown that even if a woman drinks more than just five alcoholic drinks a week, fertility-related problems could result. In the case of men, sticking to the recommended weekly alcohol allowance of 28 units is probably fine, but remember that a single big binge-drinking or drug-taking session could cause damaged sperm for the next three months. While the effects of caffeine aren't entirely clear, it would probably be beneficial for both of you to limit your daily intake to no more than one small cup of coffee or one can of caffeinated soft drink. Other environmental toxins can have strong effects on sperm too. Although this only affects a small minority of those exposed to chemicals and pesticides through their job, if this applies to you, it's worth asking your doctor whether the substances in question might be having an effect.

- **Don't overheat your testicles.** Probably the most important factor in optimizing male fertility is to make sure that your testicles don't get too warm. The reason they are outside your body in the first place is that the best temperature for good sperm production is around 3 to 4 degrees lower than your core body temperature. If you wear tight-fitting underwear or trousers or you spend the whole day sitting down, it's likely that your testicles will heat up to somewhere nearer your actual body temperature. Studies have shown that having a moderately hot bath for just 20 minutes or more could have significant effects on your sperm production. Even if your testicles get warmer by around 0.7–2.5°C (1.5–4.5°F) over regular prolonged periods, your fertility is likely to be affected. Bear in mind that the temperature of testicles will increase by up to 2.2°C (4°F) within just two hours behind the wheel of a car. Try switching to showers rather than baths and wear boxer shorts rather than tight-fitting underwear. Wear loose casual-style trousers whenever you can. Remember the three-month sperm production period means that a few major hikes in testicle temperature could have pretty long-lasting effects.

● **Get your weight right.** While for men, obesity means excess fat on the stomach and thighs, which warms up testicles and so hinders sperm production, weight is an even bigger issue for women's fertility. If you have a BMI over 25, research shows you're less likely to ovulate and more likely to suffer a miscarriage. Follow our top tips for healthy weight loss in Chapter 2 (see pages 40–2) and set yourself a time limit to lose some weight before you actively start trying to conceive. On the other hand, being underweight can have equally serious effects on fertility. Women suffering from anorexia nervosa or athletes with very low body fat sometimes stop having periods altogether. If you think about it, that's an effective defence mechanism as their bodies wouldn't have sufficient energy stores to be able to sustain a healthy pregnancy. More worryingly though, recent research at the Harvard School of Public Health has revealed that women who persistently aim for very skinny model-like bodies may be putting their fertility at serious long-term risk. The scientists found that if a woman eats a very low-fat diet over a long period of time, her brain may switch off her reproductive system altogether, although she could still continue to have periods. If your BMI is 19 or below, try to boost your weight and remember that your body does need some fat stores to work properly.

● **Get down to it.** Sometimes people forget that the best way to have a baby is to have lots of sex. It sounds obvious, but the stress of everyday life can easily impact on your sex life. Contrary to some popular myths that if you're trying to have a baby you should space out the days when you have sex to let sperm build up, the bottom line is that the more often you have sex, the greater the chance you'll get pregnant.

● **Give sperm a chance.** A man's sperm have got an arduous marathon ahead of them once they get inside a woman's body. In fact, the distance the sperm have to travel in the female reproductive system is the equivalent of 40 miles if the sperm were sized up to our proportions. They go the distance in a remarkable 15 to 20 minutes, but you can give them a hand along the way. Maximize the chance of the sperm getting to their destination by having sex that involves deep penetration (the missionary position is best, but the man behind the woman also works well). This means the semen will be ejaculated as near as possible to the woman's cervix. In positions where the woman is on top of the man or the couple are standing, the sperm are at a gravity disadvantage from the outset. What's more, after sex, the woman should try to stay lying down or even better, raise up her hips for a good 20 minutes afterwards. You could try putting your feet and legs up against the headboard or wall while you lie in bed. Don't rush off to the bathroom – even though women are advised to have a pee after sex to prevent urinary tract infections, such as cystitis, by standing up the sperm are fighting gravity by trying to swim that huge marathon upwards.

- **Know your body.** Nearly all pregnancies result from sex during the six days leading up to and ending on the day of ovulation. It's important for a woman to get to know her body's cycles: make a note of the date when your period starts and count the number of days between each one. Also look out for changes in your normal vaginal discharge. A few days before ovulation, it should become clearer and more slippery (a bit like raw egg white). If in doubt, try buying an ovulation predictor kit from a pharmacy. Don't get too hung up on having sex right at the time of ovulation – you should be having sex right across your fertile time of the month.

- **Find ways to reduce stress.** Although it's not fully understood how, your body's stress response could well be affecting your fertility. As we saw in Chapter 3 (see page 62), the stress hormone cortisol can wreak all sorts of havoc. It's believed it can interrupt the workings of the sex hormones testosterone and oestrogen, significantly affecting your chances of conceiving. If you're experiencing work or home stress, it's important you find ways to reduce it, especially if you're suffering from physical symptoms of stress, such as high blood pressure or sleep disturbances. Remember that because trying for a baby takes longer than most people imagine, that in itself can cause you to feel stressed. Check out our top tips for beating stress in Chapter 3 (see page 63) and give them a go.

- **Eat a balanced diet.** Even if you're not overweight or underweight, you could still be eating a poor diet. Your fertility is going to be at its best when your body is receiving all the proper nutrients it needs. Refer to our section on eating healthily in Chapter 1 (see page 14) and make an effort to eat well for a good few months before you actively start trying for a baby. Also, women should start taking a folic acid supplement before they aim to conceive: this has been shown to reduce substantially the number of babies born with neural tube defects, such as spina bifida (where the spine does not develop properly), particularly during the first three months of pregnancy.

- **Enjoy trying.** Few people realize before they embark on trying for a baby that it can put your relationship under an enormous amount of stress. If that happens, your sex life tends to suffer straight away – obviously not ideal if you want to get pregnant. For many people, having sex to conceive a baby can be a very different experience to having sex purely for pleasure. Give yourselves time to get used to the idea and, most importantly of all, try not to worry too much about whether or not you've conceived every time you have sex. It's important to have sex that's spontaneous and loving, rather than mechanical and timed with army precision, so give yourselves a break and remember that this is a very special time in your relationship. Within a year of regular unprotected sex, almost 90 per cent of fertile couples conceive. That figure rises to 95 per cent after two years. If you've followed all our top tips and after two years of having sex at least three or four times a week you're still not pregnant, speak to your doctor about the fertility treatments on offer.

Infertility rates – about one in six couples seek specialist help because they're having difficulty getting pregnant. Of those cases, about one-third are due to problems with the man's sperm, another third are down to problems with the woman's reproductive system and the final third remain unexplained (diagnostic tests simply fail to reveal any medical problem).

Assisted Reproductive Technology (ART) – an umbrella term to describe the myriad treatments on offer to help a couple get pregnant.

Fertility drugs – usually a first-step treatment used either to balance hormonal levels or boost a woman's fertility before trying more invasive methods.

Intrauterine Insemination (IUI) – a specially prepared sample of sperm is injected into the woman's womb at the peak time of her cycle. This may be used when the man's sperm count is low or the sperm's motility is bad, or alternatively in cases when donor sperm are used.

In Vitro Fertilization (IVF) – a procedure in which the woman takes one set of drugs to put her own reproductive system to sleep temporarily. A second drug is then used to stimulate her ovaries artificially to produce a large number of eggs. Both sets of drugs can cause side effects including depression, irritability, headaches and sleep disturbance. Once the eggs have matured, they're removed through a needle, placed in a test tube with a sperm sample from her partner and allowed to fertilize. If this happens, the embryos are then transferred back to the woman's womb (usually more than one is replaced to maximize the couple's chances of a pregnancy, but not more than three as there is then a high risk of multiple births). After two weeks, a pregnancy test establishes whether any of the embryos have successfully implanted. In the UK alone, around 24,000 couples undergo IVF each year (mostly through private clinics or assisted conception units). The success rate is around 22 per cent.

Intracytoplasmic Sperm Injection (ICSI) – a procedure that works along the same lines as IVF, but is more interventionist. Once the eggs have matured and been removed to a test tube, a single sperm is forcibly injected into the centre of an egg, using a very fine needle. The embryo is then returned to the mother, as with IVF. Success rates are much higher than IVF, although there has been some concern over possible birth defects in pregnancies achieved through ICSI, as well as the inheritance of fertility problems that otherwise would not get passed on to the next generation.

Sex selection – this is not an infertility treatment but a means of trying to produce either a male or female baby for a couple. There are various techniques available for sorting male or female sperm and also for testing the DNA of IVF-conceived embryos before transferring them back to the woman, but as yet in the UK this is only legally available for people who carry potentially serious sex-linked genetic disorders, such as Duchenne muscular dystrophy, which affects boys. In this instance, the treatment (sometimes known as pre-implantation genetic diagnosis) means a couple can be guaranteed a girl and spared the trauma of potentially having to terminate a pregnancy.

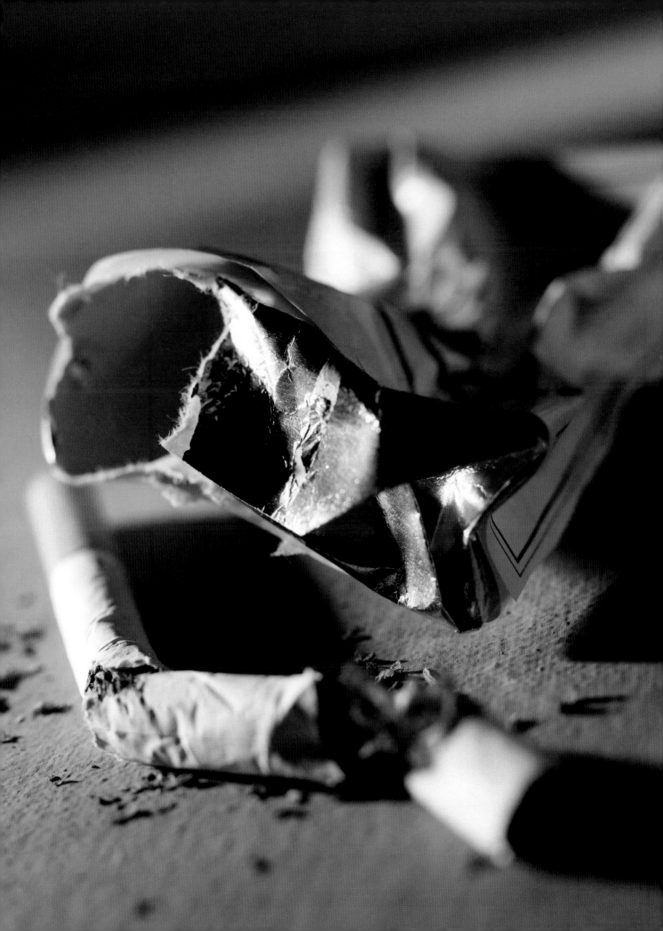

7

Avoiding Illness

In the full swing of youth, it's all too easy to feel that your body is invincible. But when the ravages of time begin to show, you're more likely to think about what lies ahead. The loss of loved ones can also make us more aware of our own health and mortality and media health scares fill the pages of our newspapers on a daily basis, provoking anxiety and confusion. But while hypochondria isn't a sensible option for anyone, knowing what illnesses you might be at risk of as time goes by and finding out how to minimize those risks will mean better health for longer – and greater peace of mind.

It's estimated that 17 million people worldwide die each year from cardio-vascular disease, particularly from heart attacks and strokes, while millions more suffering from the disease experience poor health. Each year, more than 10 million people get diagnosed with a form of cancer and 6 million die around the world. One in every three people will be diagnosed with cancer at some point during their lives. What's more, as medical advances and improved living conditions mean that life expectancy in the developed world continues to rise, we'll all be at greater risk of developing a number of chronic diseases, such as arthritis and osteoporosis, in our extended old age.

In this chapter we'll take a look at the most common forms of major illness and give you a concise capsule guide to the risk factors for each. While it's impossible to predict with any certainty which of us might succumb to major diseases in the years ahead, decades of intensive scientific research have revealed a myriad lifestyle choices that can impact on our chances. There are reams of information on all these conditions available on the Internet, but start here for the key facts, top tips and advice on lifestyle choices.

STIs – what are they?

These days, people inevitably end up having more sexual partners than they once did before settling down. While on the one hand that can result in improved sexual confidence and experience, it also leads to increasing rates of sexually transmitted infections or STIs. In Britain alone in 2002, 1.5 million people went to a genito-urinary medicine clinic with symptoms of an infection (up 15 per cent on 2001 figures).

Until the 1970s, STIs were known as venereal diseases (derived from the name of the Roman goddess of love and the Latin word for desire). However, because some of them don't produce any symptoms at all, these days they're usually more correctly referred to as sexually transmitted infections or STIs. While there are 25 different STIs out there, the main cast of contagious characters includes three bacterial infections (gonorrhoea, syphilis and chlamydia) and three viral infections (herpes simplex virus or HSV, human papilloma virus or HPV, and the dreaded HIV). There are also two infestations: pubic lice (crabs) and scabies (mites). These are tiny insects that crawl from one person to another and attach themselves firmly to coarse body hair or – in the case of scabies – burrow under the skin to lay eggs.

If you're already itching and scratching at the thought of all that, don't panic. Follow our simple symptom checklist below to find out whether or not you should get to a doctor:

STI symptoms checklist

Have you or your partner got one or more of the following?

- An unusual discharge from the vagina
- A discharge from the penis
- A burning/stinging sensation when peeing
- A rash, irritation, or swelling in the penis, vagina, testicles, or around the anus
- One or more blisters anywhere on the genital area
- Sores on the penis, vagina or anus
- Pain or bleeding after sex

Some of these symptoms can also be indicative of non-sexually transmitted medical conditions, but either way, if you have any of these symptoms, it's best to get yourself checked out. You can find details of your nearest sexual health clinic in your local telephone directory, listed under genito-urinary medicine (GUM), sexual health clinics or venereal disease clinics. In the UK, all NHS clinics provide free, confidential advice and treatment.

Understanding STIs

Here's a capsule guide to the most common STIs and how they're treated:

Parasites (pubic lice and scabies) These unwelcome guests live on coarse human hair. The most common symptom is itching in the infected areas. These insects don't really cause health problems, but they won't go away of their own accord and can spread to other hair on your body. The parasites lay their eggs in the hair follicles, so shaving won't kill them off. Mercifully, treatment is quite easy and involves two applications of a lotion or shampoo a week apart to kill off the insects and their eggs fully.

Chlamydia This is now the most common and fastest-rising bacterial STI. Data from the Health Protection Agency indicates that there were 81,680 new cases diagnosed at clinics in England, Wales and Northern Ireland in 2002 (up by 139 per cent from 1996). This

STI can be treated quite easily with a suitable course of antibiotics but do bear in mind that it's symptomless in about two-thirds of infected men and half of infected women. In some women, chlamydia spreads to the uterus and fallopian tubes and has been linked to pelvic inflammatory disease, which causes reduced fertility, ectopic pregnancy and miscarriage; and in a few men, chlamydia causes swelling in the testicles leading to infertility. All of which mean that if you're sexually active – even if you haven't got any symptoms on our

Below: Untreated chlamydia can trigger irritation and inflammation in the uterus and fallopian tubes. Pelvic Inflammatory Disease (PID) can affect ovulation, reduce fertility and lead to ectopic pregnancies.

checklist – it's well worth getting an annual sexual health check-up.

Gonorrhoea In 2002, 24,953 people in the UK were diagnosed as suffering from this bacterial infection (over double that recorded in 1996). A burning, stinging sensation when peeing coupled with a nasty discharge from the penis or vagina is the likely signature of gonorrhoea. Like chlamydia, it needs to be treated early and can cause pelvic inflammatory disease in women. In the past, this was successfully treated with penicillin but now several resistant strains have emerged, so new antibiotics or combinations of medications are often prescribed. Usually a single treatment with a follow-up test is all that is needed.

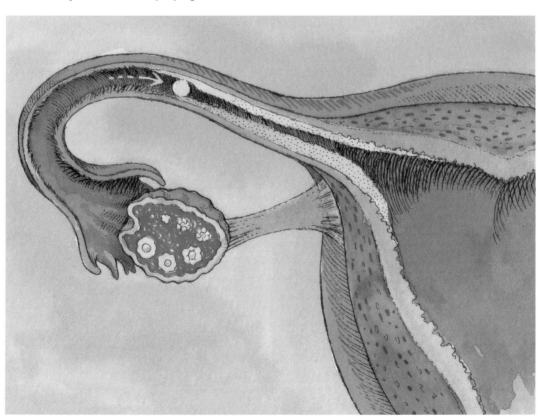

Syphilis The calling card of syphilis is a single painful blister turning into an ulcerated sore on the penis, vagina, anus or mouth. Back in the early 1990s, there were signs that we had eradicated this nasty STI. But in the UK in 2002, 1193 new cases were reported, which represented an alarming 63 per cent increase on 2001 and a staggering 870 per cent increase on 1996. Of the cases in 2002, 51 per cent were thought to be due to male homosexual activity, and major and sustained outbreaks of syphilis infection were recorded in London and Manchester. If left untreated, the syphilis sore will disappear but can eventually lead to a cluster of very unpleasant circulatory, cardiovascular and neurological problems. Fortunately,

treatment isn't too difficult and penicillin remains the most common medication prescribed.

Genital herpes Genital herpes infections are caused by the herpes simplex virus (type II). The major symptoms of HSV are one or more small, highly infectious blisters in the genital area, and sometimes around the mouth, which burst to leave painful sores. After a first major outbreak, during which the sufferer can feel pretty unwell (a headache and swollen

Below: The herpes simplex virus (HSV) causes painful and highly infectious sores in the genital area, but is also connected to cold sores that appear around the mouth. The infection is lifelong and periodic outbreaks are common.

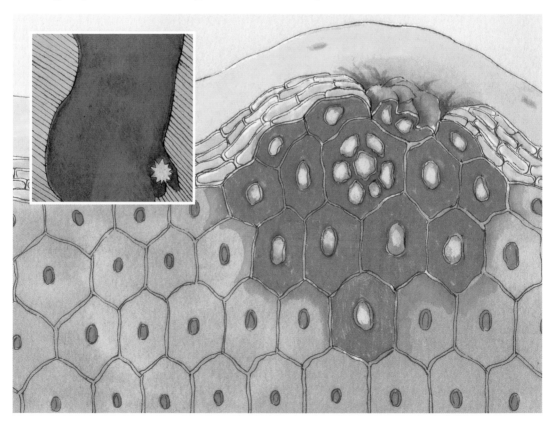

glands are sometimes experienced), the sores gradually dry out and disappear over the next month but then usually reappear from time to time. The sores themselves can be calmed with an antiviral treatment. Although there are no long-term serious health problems, genital herpes infections last for life.

Genital warts The incidence of genital wart infection is very common all over the world. The warts are caused by the human papilloma virus or HPV and are usually small, hard white/pinkish bumps on the genital area or around the anus and can grow to take on a more irregular, cauliflower-like appearance. They can be itchy and irritating. Bear in mind that some types of HPV are thought to increase the risk of cervical cancer in women, so do get any genital warts treated. This is usually successful but wart outbreaks can reoccur. A clinic will prescribe a topical anti-wart liquid or cream to be applied directly; in some cases larger genital warts may need to be removed by freezing them off.

HIV/AIDS HIV is a retrovirus that progressively weakens the body's ability to fight infections and can eventually lead to AIDS. Infection usually triggers an initial flu-like illness, then most people live without major symptoms for a decade before suffering from a major illness that results in their death. Latest estimates suggest that 42 million people around the world are currently infected with HIV. There were 3342 new cases diagnosed in the UK in 2001. Since 1999, the number of new cases of HIV acquired through heterosexual sex has outnumbered those acquired through men having sex with men. Although HIV remains incurable, modern combination antiretroviral

treatment has achieved remarkable results in keeping people healthy for longer.

Protect yourself

Unsurprisingly, the most common route of STI transmission is through unprotected genital contact with the surface of infected skin. But few people realize that some bacteria or viruses can also be passed during oral sex and an infection can even occasionally be transferred on fingers from the genitals to the mouth or eyes. Even something as innocent as kissing can transfer the genital herpes virus if a partner has active sores on their mouth.

The best strategy to protect yourself is to use a condom when you have sex. Research shows that consistent condom use reduces the risk of HIV transmission by 85 per cent. However, condoms sometimes do break or slip off. Recent US research indicates that condom failure rates due to breakage or slippage (during sex or at withdrawal) are between 1.6 and 3.6 per cent. Buying condoms that are the right size, putting them on properly and using lubricant all bring the failure rate down. But you should also bear in mind that even if you do use a condom, other parts of your genital area may still come into direct contact with your partner's, which means you could still contract herpes (HSV) and genital warts (HPV).

Remember that the more sexual partners you have – even if you are having safe sex or you've had a series of long-term relationships rather than one-night stands – the higher your chance of picking up an STI. Use condoms to minimize that risk and keep a close eye on your sexual health so that you can get any infections treated as quickly as possible before they affect your health or you pass them on.

Heart disease – what is it?

Coronary heart disease starts when fatty deposits laid down on the inside of your arteries cause them to become narrow and impede blood flow. At this stage, the condition is called atherosclerosis but as it progresses, the fatty deposits become such an obstruction that insufficient amounts of blood get through to the heart muscle and it gets deprived of oxygen. That's when angina develops, causing pain in your chest or arm – usually when you're exerting yourself physically and so the heart is under more pressure. The serious problems begin if a blood clot happens to block a narrowed artery and if that happens in a coronary artery, you'd have a heart attack. Blockages in other types of blood vessels could lead to an ischaemic attack or a stroke.

What causes it?

Although heart disease tends to run in families, and there are probably several genes that predispose you to laying down fat in your arteries, there are four key lifestyle factors that have been shown to exacerbate heart disease:

A bad diet – eating an unhealthy diet can drastically affect the health of your heart. Your liver produces a substance called cholesterol, which helps all your body's cells to work healthily. It's transported around your body in two forms: LDL (low-density lipoprotein), which carries cholesterol from your liver to all your cells and HDL (high-density lipoprotein), which returns excess cholesterol to your liver. Almost all the cholesterol in your body is made by your liver breaking down the saturated fats you've consumed in food – the more fat you eat, the higher your LDL levels rise and the lower your HDL levels fall. LDL is the baddie of the story – it's responsible for those fatty deposits inside arteries – while HDL seems to have a protective effect on your heart. In addition, if you eat a high-fat diet, you're far more likely to be overweight or obese, which can put your heart under even greater strain and raise your blood pressure.

Smoking cigarettes – two of the main chemicals in cigarette smoke, carbon monoxide and nicotine, wreak havoc on your heart. Carbon monoxide hijacks a special protein called haemoglobin, which is responsible for carrying oxygen around your body in your blood. If you're a smoker, your heart could be getting as little as half the oxygen it needs to function properly. Nicotine makes your body produce adrenaline, which raises your blood pressure and makes your heart work harder.

Having high blood pressure – if you suffer from high blood pressure (also known as hypertension), you are at much greater risk of experiencing a heart attack or stroke. It is worth getting your blood pressure checked out as even if it's high – the chances are you won't experience any particular symptoms. You may be predisposed to hypertension, or it could have resulted from a number of different factors: being overweight, suffering high levels of stress, eating too much salt or drinking too much alcohol.

Being inactive – exercising regularly – or even just being physically active – has been shown to improve the health of your heart. It seems to increase levels of the good cholesterol (HDL), which counteracts the effects of the bad stuff (LDL). It also regulates blood pressure, helps you keep to a healthy weight and stop blood clots from forming.

Are you at risk of heart disease?

If you're worried about whether your lifestyle might be damaging your heart and arteries, answer the following questions (to answer questions 5 and 6 you need to have had some simple tests done by your doctor):

1 Do you smoke?
YES/NO

2 Are you overweight?
Refer to page 34 to find out how to work out your body mass index (BMI).
YES/NO

3 Do you feel you could be more physically active?
YES/NO

4 Has anyone in your close family died of coronary heart disease, a heart attack or a stroke?
YES/NO

5 Is your blood pressure higher than 140/85?
YES/NO

6 Is your LDL cholesterol level higher than 3 mmol/l or your total cholesterol over 5 mmol/l?
YES/NO

If you answered yes to questions 1, 2 or 3, you can make some simple changes to your lifestyle to improve your heart health – follow our advice on pages 134–5.

If you answered yes to questions 4, 5 or 6, your risk of cardiovascular disease is higher and as well as insuring you follow our tips on pages 134–5, you need to consult your doctor regularly so your heart can be monitored.

Top tips for a healthy heart

Below are some straightforward steps you can take to improve your lifestyle. Not all of them are easy and they may well require some willpower and determination, but bear in mind that all these tips should improve your overall health and wellbeing, so it's worth making the effort.

- **Give up smoking.** You can halve your risk of a heart attack within five years of giving up smoking – not to mention your risk of a whole host of other serious diseases, such as lung, mouth and throat cancer. Try everything you can to give up, be it nicotine patches, gum, or even hypnosis. If you're finding it tough, speak to your doctor for more advice.

- **What about just cutting down?** It's true that the more cigarettes you smoke, the greater your risk of a heart attack, but smoking less doesn't stop those harmful chemicals from affecting your body. Even 24 hours after your last cigarette, there'll be the same amount of carbon monoxide inside you. Likewise, don't be fooled by 'light', 'mild' or 'low-tar' cigarettes. They may indeed have less tar, which may marginally reduce the chance of cancer, but that doesn't mean the amount of carbon monoxide and nicotine have been reduced – in other words, low-tar cigarettes are just as damaging to your heart.

- **Eat less salt.** Eating more than 6 grams of salt a day is likely to cause hikes in your blood pressure. Try to cut down or consider swapping to reduced-salt or low-salt brands. Never add salt to your food without tasting it first and be aware that most processed foods contain very high amounts of salt. Start

checking food labels before you buy. If food tastes too bland without salt, try adding herbs and spices instead.

- **Eat fewer saturated fats.** Cutting down on saturated fats found in red meat, fried foods, cakes, sweets, crisps and full-fat dairy products will help you keep to a healthy weight too, which should lower your blood pressure.

- **Ditch dangerous fats.** Replace bad fats with monounsaturated fats, such as olive oil, or polyunsaturated fats, such as sunflower oil – but make sure you still only eat them in small amounts.

- **Eat more fish.** Research has shown that some fish contain an oil called omega-3, which can improve your heart health, if eaten regularly. Try trout, anchovies, sardines, pilchards, kippers or herring or tuna. If you don't fancy fish, consider taking a fish oil or cod liver oil supplement every day.

- **Eat more fruit and vegetables.** Eat at least five portions of fruit and vegetables each day – they've been shown to inhibit fatty deposits being laid down in your arteries, improve your blood pressure and reduce levels of an amino acid in your body called homocysteine (which is known to increase the levels of LDL cholesterol in your arteries). People who have heart disease often have high levels of homocysteine so it's worth keeping a lid on it.

- **Exercise.** Include more physical activity in your daily life: walk instead of driving or taking public transport and try the stairs instead of a lift or elevator. Make sure you're active enough that you get slightly breathless – that way you know your heart is getting a workout. If you can include a moderate amount of exercise in your life on a regular basis, your heart will reap the benefits. Not only that, but you should be able to keep your weight within a healthy range and keep your blood pressure down too. Reducing your blood pressure by even just a small amount can reduce your risk of having a heart attack by up to 20 per cent.

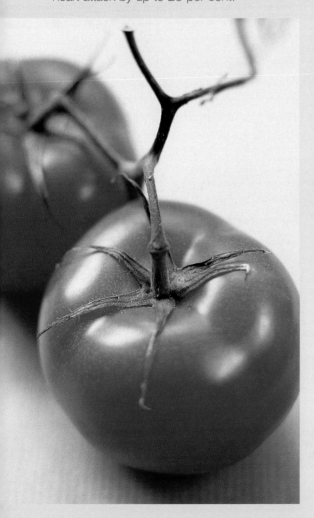

- **Drink less alcohol.** It's fine to drink moderately and responsibly, but anything above the maximum recommended weekly units of alcohol (21 units for women and 28 units for men) could be raising your blood pressure and putting your heart under extra strain. Binge-drinking in particular is thought to be a key culprit of heart disease. Look at our section on drinking in Chapter 1 (see pages 21–31) for more information on what constitutes a unit of alcohol and how you can cut down on your intake.

- **Women beware.** You might think of heart disease as something that usually affects men, but after the menopause your risk of developing it is just as high. The female sex hormone oestrogen helps to protect you during your fertile years (by laying fat down on your hips and thighs, where it can't do too much damage to your heart or coronary arteries). After the menopause, when oestrogen levels drop drastically, you're more likely to put fat on around your waist as men do, which will put your heart under far greater strain.

- **Be aware.** Make sure you keep an eye on your blood pressure and if you feel you're at high risk of heart disease for whatever reason, your cholesterol should be checked regularly too. Over-the-counter cholesterol tests are an indicator but they won't be as reliable as the type you can have done by your doctor.

Left: Fruit and vegetables keep your heart healthy, so make sure they're part of your daily diet.

Cancer – what is it?

Cancer develops when a group of cells anywhere in your body starts multiplying and growing out of control. This creates a tumour, which can then spread to other tissues or organs in your body. Ten million people around the world get diagnosed with a form of cancer each year.

What causes it?

Cancerous cells develop when the genes that make cells work healthily in the first place get damaged. You might carry genes that predispose you to this happening or you may be exposing yourself to lifestyle risks that significantly increase your chances of developing a certain type of cancer. As you get older, so your chances of getting cancer increase – most cancers affect those over the age of 65. But as you'll see below, there's plenty you can do to try and optimize your chances of staying healthy. In fact, it's now believed that as many as one-third of cancers could be prevented through lifestyle changes.

Could it be cancer?

While medical advances have vastly improved the survival chances of people with cancer, the key to recovery still lies in early detection of the condition. It's important to keep a regular, watchful check on the health of your body without becoming too anxious or obsessed about your chances of developing cancer. Look at the checklist opposite to work out whether or not it's worth a visit to your doctor.

What can you do?

If one of your close relatives (that is a parent, sibling, child, grandparent, aunt, uncle, niece or nephew) has been diagnosed with or has died from a type of cancer, it would be worth you finding out some more information about it, if you haven't already. That's not to say that all cancers are hereditary by any means, but you could be at greater risk of developing them yourself in years to come. Check information from local cancer research and support organizations and speak to your doctor to find out more about your situation. Below are capsule guides to the most common forms of cancer you may be concerned about: lung, colon, breast, cervical, testicular and prostate, including specific advice for checking yourself for symptoms and changing your lifestyle to reduce the risk of developing each one.

However, there are six simple, key pieces of advice that apply to the vast majority of cancers (see page 138). If you can make the effort to fit these into your lifestyle, your risk of developing cancer should be significantly reduced.

Read on for the key facts on some of the most common cancers:

Lung cancer

● Smoking causes 90 per cent of lung cancer cases.

● Passive smoking counts too: if you live with a smoker, your chances of getting lung cancer are much higher than if you live in a smoke-free environment.

● One person dies of lung cancer every 15 minutes in the UK.

● There were nearly 250,000 new cases of lung cancer diagnosed in Europe in 2000.

● Nicotine itself isn't carcinogenic, just highly addictive. Once you've got a habit,

Cancer checklist

Have you noticed any of the following:

1 **Any unexpected bleeding from any part of your body or in your bowel movements or urine?**
YES/NO

2 **A lump anywhere on your body?**
YES/NO

3 **Ongoing pain or discomfort that you can't explain?**
YES/NO

4 **Weight loss that you can't explain?**
YES/NO

5 **Any unusual change in your bowel habits?**
YES/NO

6 **A persistent cough or difficulty breathing or swallowing?**
YES/NO

7 **A mole that has changed in shape, size or colour, is itchy or bleeds?**
YES/NO

If you answered yes to any of the above, don't panic. It doesn't necessarily mean that you've got cancer, but it's important that you get yourself checked out by a doctor as soon as possible. If you've answered no to all the questions, keep these general symptoms in mind and remember to make an appointment with your doctor if you ever experience any of them.

Six top tips for preventing cancer

1 Stop smoking. Although lung cancer is most commonly associated with cigarettes, smoking is also linked to cancer of the gullet (or oesophagus), throat and mouth and perhaps more surprisingly, cancer of the pancreas, bladder, liver, cervix, kidney and stomach.

2 Eat a healthy diet. If you can stick to a healthy weight and eat a good, balanced diet, you'll be protecting yourself against cancer of the gullet, stomach, colon, pancreas, breast, lung, prostate and bladder. All the more reason to cut down on sugars, saturated fats and salt and eat more fibre and fruit and vegetables every day. Refer to Chapter 1 (see page 14) if you need more advice.

3 Drink less. High intake of alcohol has been shown to increase your risk of developing cancer of the mouth, throat and gullet. There's also evidence to suggest that breast, liver and colon cancer may be linked to drinking too much alcohol. Stick to the recommended limits (see page 27) and avoid binge-drinking.

4 Exercise. Keeping fit helps you to maintain a healthy weight and keep your overall health up to scratch. Try exercising moderately or even just being very physically active for at least half an hour three times a week. Make sure that the physical activity is strenuous enough to make you slightly breathless, so that your heart gets the exercise it needs.

5 Keep safe when you're out and about. Protect your skin from the sun's radiation. Wear a hat, sit in the shade and if you do expose your skin to the sun, wear a high SPF sun protection cream of at least 25. Check out our advice in Chapter 4 (see pages 83–5) for more information on how to be safe in the sun. If your working environment involves you being exposed to asbestos, radiation or any strong chemicals, be sure to follow health and safety regulations to the letter and if you're concerned, ask your doctor for extra advice.

6 Check yourself and get checked. It's important to keep an eye on your body's health whenever you can. See our advice on pages 142 and 145 on examining your breasts or testicles and make sure you follow your doctor's advice on screening tests, so that you always keep up to date on cervical smears (pap tests) or mammograms, if you need them.

carbon monoxide hampers your breathing and you'll be inhaling a regular high dose of tar, which is known to cause cancer.

- The more cigarettes you smoke, the greater your risk of lung cancer.

- If you give up before the age of 35, your life expectancy shouldn't be that different from non-smokers.

- Your risk of getting cancer starts to decrease as soon as you give up. Once you've given up for ten years, your risk of lung cancer is halved and after 15 years, your chances of developing the disease are almost identical to someone who's never smoked at all.

- Low-tar cigarettes or those labelled as 'light' or 'mild' can be very misleading. While they appear to contain less carcinogenic tar, research has shown that smokers of low-tar cigarettes tend to inhale much more deeply without even realizing it, so that they get a high enough dose to achieve the same nicotine kick.

Protect yourself against lung cancer

- There's just one piece of advice that will give you drastically increased protection against lung cancer: give up smoking altogether. It's tough to quit because nicotine is a highly addictive drug, but there are many ways you can try. Refer to our 'quit smoking' section in Chapter 8 (see page 154). Don't be put off if you've tried to give up unsuccessfully in the past – with help and support you can do it. Speak to your doctor, a local support group or a telephone helpline for advice.

Colon cancer

- This is also known as bowel or colorectal cancer.

- Abnormal cells amass into a small growth called a polyp anywhere in the colon or rectum. While this can remain benign, it can also develop into a cancerous tumour and spread out of the bowel to other parts of the body, usually the liver.

- The first symptoms of a problem tend to be blood or mucus in your bowel movements. Any unusual change in your bowel habits can also signify a problem. In most cases, bleeding will simply be down to haemorrhoids (piles), but if over-the-counter pile creams don't seem to be working after a short while, get yourself checked out by a doctor as soon as possible, so you can be sure it's nothing more serious. If there is a possibility of cancer, the longer you leave it, the more your chances of successful treatment are reduced.

- There were nearly 260,000 new cases diagnosed in Europe in 2000.

- 90 per cent of people who develop colon cancer are over the age of 50.

- If a person develops colon cancer before the age of 40, there's a greater chance that a genetic predisposition is involved.

- Eating a lot of fibre in your diet helps to protect you against colon cancer, although no-one knows for sure why this is. One possible explanation is that if you don't eat enough fibre you can get constipated, which means all the waste matter in your colon takes much longer to move through it. This might give potentially risky substances more time to damage cells in your bowel.

● High-fibre fruit and vegetables also seem to keep cells properly nourished with vitamin and mineral nutrients, which means they have less chance of being damaged and turning cancerous.

Protect yourself against colon cancer

● As well as adapting your diet to include less sugar, saturated fat and salt as we discussed earlier in the chapter, make sure you eat a good daily dose of naturally fibre-rich foods, such as wholegrain cereals, beans, pulses, fruit and vegetables. Remember five portions a day is a good minimum guideline for the amount of fruit and vegetables you should be eating.

● Eat more vegetables rich in folic acid. Try including more spinach, asparagus, avocado, broccoli and cabbage in your diet.

● Bear in mind that studies show the risk of bowel cancer is 50 per cent lower in those who exercise regularly.

● Although we're brought up to think of toilet matters as embarrassing, it's vital to keep an eye on your bowel movements for traces of blood, mucus or any change in your usual habits, so that if you do develop bowel cancer, it's detected as early as possible. It could save your life, so make it a daily habit.

Right: A healthy diet can still be a tasty one and will help protect you against illness and disease.

Breast cancer

● One out of every nine women will develop breast cancer at some point during their lifetime.

● The risk rises dramatically once you reach the age of 50.

● 80 per cent of cases of breast cancer in the UK occur in post-menopausal women. Your risk of the disease increases significantly with age.

● In 2000, there were nearly 380,000 deaths from breast cancer around the world and nearly 250,000 new cases of the disease diagnosed in Europe.

● The more children you've had and the younger you were when you had them, the smaller your chances are of developing breast cancer.

● If you breast-fed your children, your risk of breast cancer is also reduced. This is possibly due to the fact that during breast-feeding, the female body doesn't ovulate, so overall it's exposed to less of the female hormone oestrogen than non-breastfeeding mothers or non-childbearing women.

● It's known that the female hormone oestrogen encourages the growth of breast tumours, so taking the contraceptive pill (which contains oestrogen) may increase your risk of breast cancer very slightly. However, as most users are in their twenties or thirties and therefore not at high risk of the disease anyway, it shouldn't make too much difference. Studies show that ten years after coming off the pill women are at no greater risk than non-users. On the plus side, the

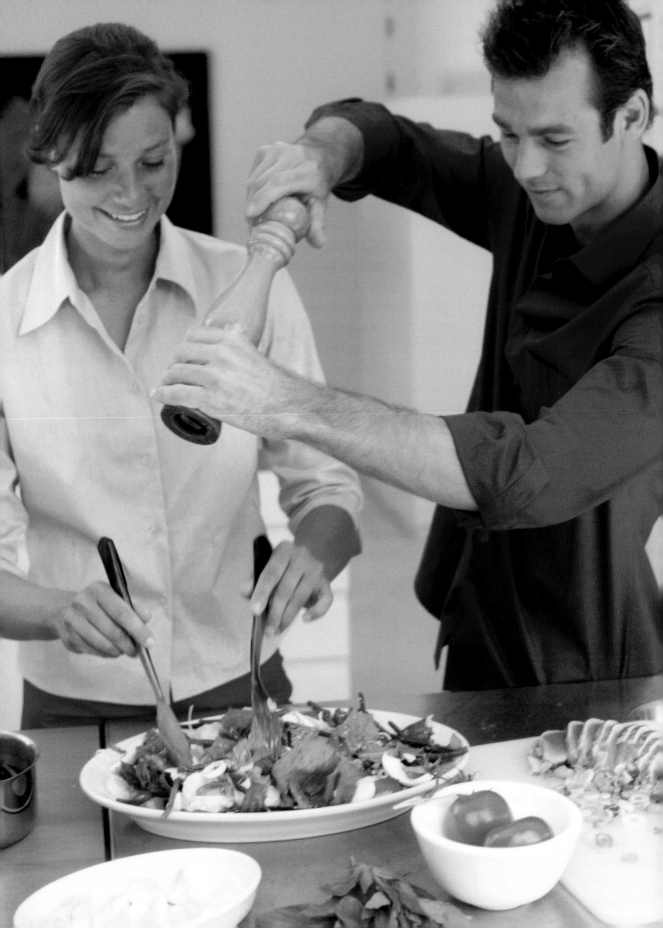

contraceptive pill does appear to offer some protection against both cancer of the ovary and of the uterus.

● Hormone replacement therapy (HRT) carries a possible breast cancer risk, especially as women who take it tend to be in the post-menopausal age group, and are therefore more at risk of developing breast cancer anyway. There's evidence to suggest that combined HRT (which contains both oestrogen and progesterone) is more likely to cause breast cancer than oestrogen-only HRT. There is also an increased risk of heart disease with HRT, although there's evidence that it may protect against some forms of colon cancer and the bone disease osteoporosis.

● A small number of women carry rare genes that are known to increase their chances of developing breast cancer. There are currently tests available to screen for two of these genes, BRCA1 and BRCA2. If one or more of your close relatives (which means your mother, sister, daughter, grandmother, aunt or niece) has been diagnosed with breast cancer under the age of 50, it would be worth discussing genetic screening tests with your doctor, if you haven't already. Don't panic too much though – experts believe that only 5 per cent of breast cancer cases are due to a known genetic cause.

● If you're a woman aged between 50 and 64 and you live in the UK, you should be having a mammogram (breast x-ray) once every three years, as part of the breast cancer screening programme run by the NHS. If you're not up to date, book an appointment with your doctor – it could save your life.

Protect yourself against breast cancer

● **Examine your breasts** – no matter what your age, you can start protecting yourself against breast cancer by keeping vigilant. Get to know your breasts; it's important that you check them regularly, say once a month at least. That way you can get a good idea of what is normal for you and whether or not any changes have occurred. Pre-menstrual hormonal changes can cause swelling and discomfort in the breasts, so the best time to check them is after your period when they've settled down again. Keep a look-out for any of the following:

1 A lump or swelling in one of your breasts, nipples or armpits.
2 Any dimpling or puckering in the breasts or nipples.
3 Any changes in size or shape of your breasts or nipples.
4 Any discharge from your nipples.
5 Unusual pains or aches in your breasts (although bear in mind that it's normal to feel some tenderness in your breasts at different times in your menstrual cycle).

● **Ask your doctor's advice** – if you find something unusual, try not to panic as 90 per cent of breast lumps aren't actually cancerous. You may just have a cyst or a benign lump. Either way, it's imperative that you go to the doctor to get it checked out as soon as possible, as survival chances for breast cancer rise dramatically if it's detected early.

● **Drink less alcohol** – studies have shown that drinking over the recommended limit of 21 units a week puts women at greater risk of breast cancer. If you're taking HRT, consider drinking even less – no more than 14 units a week. Refer to Chapter 1 (see pages 21–31) for information on what constitutes a unit and how you can go about cutting down.

Cervical cancer

● There are 370,000 new cases of cervical cancer around the world each year.

● Organized screening programmes have resulted in a decrease in mortality in this disease by as much as 60 per cent.

● If you're a sexually active woman living in the UK and you're aged between 21 and 64, you should be having a regular cervical smear or pap test as part of the cervical cancer screening programme run by the NHS. (The test involves taking a cell sample from the cervix, which sits at the top of the inside of a woman's vagina.) You'll be called for a smear test every three or five years, depending on the screening policy in your local area.

● Cervical cancer is a slow-developing disease. A cluster of cells on the cervix will become abnormal and go through some 'pre-cancerous' stages before finally developing into a tumour. Once again, early detection offers the best chances of recovery and survival.

● Symptoms can include pain during or after sex and bleeding at times other than during your period. However, you may also have no symptoms at all. If you do experience pain or abnormal bleeding, don't panic as these don't necessarily mean you've got cancer, but you should have them checked out by a doctor as soon as possible.

● As we discussed in our section on sexually transmitted infections (STIs) – see pages 128–31 – one of the main risk factors for developing cervical cancer is being exposed to the human papilloma virus (HPV). There are more than 100 different strains of this virus, most of which are transmitted through unprotected sex. Some types of HPV are responsible for genital warts, but these strains aren't generally linked with cervical cancer. However, there are more than a dozen types of HPV that are believed to trigger the disease.

● If you've been infected with the potentially cancer-causing strains of HPV, you're unlikely to have any symptoms, nor is the virus curable. However, only a small number of women infected with HPV will go on to develop cervical cancer. Nevertheless, because HPV is very common, it's extremely important to always attend cervical smears so that any changes in the cells of your cervix can be picked up as soon as possible.

● Smoking has also been shown to be a direct risk factor for cervical cancer. Researchers have even found traces of carcinogenic chemicals from cigarettes in the cervical mucus of some female smokers. It's known that these compounds damage special cells in your cervix that normally repair cells there if they become abnormal.

● Taking the oral contraceptive pill is also believed to increase your risk of cervical cancer slightly. It's possible that this is also a reflection of the fact that women on the pill are more likely to be sexually active and unlikely to be using a barrier method of contraception, so their chances of being exposed to HPV are much higher. However, don't panic too much as the increase in risk isn't that great: nine out of every thousand non-pill-using women will go on to develop cervical cancer, whereas it's estimated that ten out of each thousand pill-taking women will go on to develop the disease. That risk does increase if you take the pill for long periods of time (18 women out of every thousand who take the pill for more than ten years will get cervical cancer). The good news is that by having regular smears much of that extra risk gets cancelled out.

Protect yourself against cervical cancer

● **Use a condom** – if you're sexually active, bear in mind that the more sexual partners you have, the greater your chances of being exposed to cancer-causing strains of HPV. To protect yourself the best strategy is always to ask your partner to wear a condom.

● **Make sure your partner has a good level of hygiene** – if you're in a long-term relationship and would prefer to use a non-barrier method of contraception, for instance the pill, make sure that your partner regularly washes his penis and in particular the foreskin area if he's not circumsized. Washing before and after sex is a good idea.

● **Go for regular cervical smears (or pap tests)** – your doctor should remind you when these need to be done. They are slightly uncomfortable but could well save your life.

● **Give up smoking** – studies show that if you smoke, you're more likely to get HPV and if you're infected with a cancer-causing strain of HPV and are still smoking, your chances of developing cervical cancer are higher. Refer to our 'quit smoking' section in Chapter 8 (see page 154) for further advice on how to go about giving up cigarettes.

Testicular cancer

● This is the most common form of cancer in men aged between 15 and 45 – in fact, it is one of the few cancers for which the risk begins to fall for men over the age of 45.

● Its incidence is still quite rare (around 2000 cases are diagnosed in the UK each year). However, it is believed that worldwide rates of the disease have risen significantly over the last few decades.

● Cancerous cells start proliferating in one of the testicles and may spread to the lymph glands near the back or pelvis. If left to progress, the cancer could spread to other organs, usually the lungs.

● Men who have an undescended testicle or any kind of testicle abnormality are at greater risk of developing the disease.

● Men with fertility problems have also been shown to be more likely to get testicular cancer, although the risk is raised only slightly.

● It's believed that if your testicles repeatedly suffer a rise in temperature brought on by always wearing tight underwear or trousers, or even by a very sedentary lifestyle, there may be an increased risk.

● Experts think that as many as 20 per cent of cases of testicular cancer could be down to a few inherited faulty genes. They've already identified one culprit (known as TGCT1), which is inherited from the man's mother on the X chromosome. That's why brothers sometimes both suffer the disease.

Protect yourself against testicular cancer

● **Check your testicles** – although testicular cancer is usually extremely treatable and has a high survival rate, early detection is once again the key to recovery. Whatever your age, you should make sure you check your testicles on a regular basis. Because testicular cancer rarely occurs in both testicles, it's worth comparing anything you think is unusual in one testicle to the other. Look out for any of the following:

1 Any change in size or shape of either testicle.
2 Aching or discomfort in either testicle.
3 A painless swelling or lump in a testicle.
4 A heavy feeling in your scrotum.

● **Seek advice from your doctor** – if you experience any of the above symptoms, try not to panic. The vast majority of testicular lumps turn out not to be cancer, but it's vital you see a doctor as soon as possible to get a clean bill of health.

Prostate cancer

● In 2000 there were half a million new cases of prostate cancer reported worldwide, and around 204,000 men died from the disease.

● The vast majority of cases of prostate cancer (around 80 per cent) occur in men who are over the age of 50.

● In the UK, one man in every 14 will develop the disease at some stage in his life.

● This form of cancer is very slow-growing. However, if it progresses it's likely to spread to the lymph nodes and bones in the hip and lower back.

● Prostate cancer cases have risen over the last few years, but experts put that down to the fact that screening programmes have revealed more cases of the disease. Doctors can check the health of your prostate gland by testing your blood for a special substance called prostate specific antigen (PSA), which is produced by the gland. If your PSA levels are high, this may simply indicate an infection or inflammation in your prostate. However, elevated levels over a number of tests might reflect something more serious.

● The walnut-sized prostate surrounds the urethra (the tube which runs from your bladder) and adds fluid to sperm when a man ejaculates. When a man urinates, the bladder will be emptied straight down the urethra through his penis, but during ejaculation, the prostate squeezes the urethra shut to stop urine from mixing with semen. If the prostate gland swells up for whatever reason, you might experience blocked urine flow or other urinary problems.

● An inflamed or infected prostate is quite common as men get older. Although it is relatively harmless, it will produce many of the same symptoms as prostate cancer. If you notice a more frequent need to urinate, especially at night, difficulty, pain or discomfort when you urinate or traces of blood in your urine or semen, it's important to get yourself checked out by a doctor as soon as you can.

Protect yourself against prostate cancer

● **Keep an eye on your urinary health** – even if you're a man under the age of 50, it's important to track any changes that occur as

Top tips for protecting your joints

- **Keep to a healthy weight.** Being overweight or obese puts much more strain on your joints, which could add to wear and tear on them as you get older.

- **Eat plenty of fruit and vegetables.** Yet another reason to consume at least five portions of these a day – they're rich in all manner of vitamins and anti-oxidants that help to keep your joints healthy.

- **Avoid joint injury.** If your job involves lots of physical activity, heavy lifting or even just repetitive movements, such as typing, make sure your joints get good periods of rest now and again. If joint pain develops and you just put it down to tiredness, consider speaking to your employers about how you could limit strain injuries by changing your working practice.

- **Don't overdo it.** If you take part in sports that involve impact on your joints or you exercise regularly, be sure to always include a warm-up period and carry out stretching exercises after your workout. If you ever feel pain or discomfort, give your body a rest and don't resume your exercise or sports programme until you're fully recovered. That said, bear in mind that high levels of physical inactivity actually increase your risk of osteoarthritis as joints can seize up through under-use, so do exercise regularly, just don't overdo it.

the years go by. Men are often unwilling to see a doctor about what they consider to be mild urinary symptoms, but remember that early detection is essential for good levels of recovery and survival in cases of prostate cancer, so it's always best to get yourself checked out by a doctor.

- **Eat plenty of tomatoes** – as well as keeping to a healthy diet as we've described earlier (see page 14), make sure you eat plenty of tomatoes. They contain high amounts of a substance called lycopene. Studies of men who eat a lycopene-rich diet suggest they have a greatly reduced risk of prostate cancer.

- **Be extra vigilant** – if one of your close male relatives (that is your grandfather, father or a brother) has been diagnosed with prostate cancer, you should be extra careful about the health of your prostate. You might even consider having a regular PSA test as you get older. Speak to your doctor for further advice on your situation.

Thinking ahead about illness

As we mentioned earlier, increased life expectancy all over the developed world means that in years to come, all of us will be at greater risk of developing some of the chronic and debilitating diseases of old age. While your elderly years may well be a long way off, it's worth bearing in mind that there are quite a few lifestyle steps you can take now to help improve your chances of preventing certain diseases, such as arthritis, osteoporosis and Alzheimer's disease developing when you're older. Such conditions might seem irrelevant to you right now, but this is a key time to take action and protect your future health.

Arthritis – what is it?

This is a group of conditions in which the action of one or more of the moving joints in your body becomes painful and difficult. Each of your joints is made up of two moving bone surfaces that are cushioned by a layer of cartilage and a fluid-filled sac, which enable healthy joints to move smoothly and comfortably. Arthritis occurs when either the cartilage, the fluid (known as synovial fluid) or its thin membranous sac become damaged. If you've ever known someone who suffers from arthritis, you'll know it can be an extremely painful and distressing condition – one to be avoided if at all possible.

What causes it?

There are many different causes for arthritis. Experts believe that in its most common form, osteoarthritis, there could be a number of culprits to blame. Joint over-use, under-use, injury or simply age bring about a joint inflammation and degeneration that eventually leads to the cartilage being worn away and the underlying bones being exposed. This tends to be particularly painful and debilitating when it occurs in weight-bearing joints, such as the hip. It's estimated that more than 100 million people around the world suffer from osteoarthritis, with almost all cases developing after the age of 45.

Top tips for protecting your bones

- **Get your calcium.** Bones need calcium to help them grow and stay strong. You should be getting 700 mg of calcium each day from your food. Eat plenty of dairy products, such as milk or cheese, or you can also get your calcium by eating lots of leafy vegetables, for example spinach or watercress, as well as oily fish, for instance pilchards and sardines. Two hundred millilitres (7 fl oz) of semi-skimmed milk gives you around 230 mg of calcium, while a slice of wholemeal bread contains 16 mg. You'd need to eat about 100 g (3½ oz) of boiled spinach to get 160 mg of calcium. Keep an eye out for cereals and grains that are calcium-enriched. But don't overdo it as excessive consumption of calcium can cause medical problems. Check what amount of it you're getting from your daily multi-vitamin supplement, if you take one, but bear in mind that almost all varieties of these don't give you enough to reach the recommended daily limit, so you should make up the remainder through your diet.

- **Eat plenty of fruit and vegetables.** A healthy, balanced diet will make an important contribution to your bone health as the years go by.

- **Exercise regularly.** Moderate amounts of weight-bearing exercise have been shown to keep bones in good condition. Try walking at a fast pace, running or even scaling the stairs on a regular basis.

- **Give up smoking.** Studies have shown that harmful chemicals in cigarettes damage the condition of your bones – in fact, it's estimated that one in eight hip fractures occur in people who have weakened bones as a result of smoking.

Osteoporosis – what is it?

Inside all your bones is a strong, mesh-like tissue – remarkably, your bone tissue gets completely renewed every ten years or so. But as you age, that thick mesh of bone cells, proteins and minerals (particularly calcium) becomes thinner and weaker. Osteoporosis is a condition in which the bones are literally porous and so much more liable to break, even in relatively minor falls or trips. Worldwide, one in three women and one in eight men over the age of 50 are affected. Every three minutes, osteoporosis causes someone in the UK to break a bone. Because the female sex hormone oestrogen helps in the process of regenerating bone cells, women are particularly at risk after the menopause, when oestrogen levels drop dramatically.

What causes it?

During your youth, your bones are constantly growing and strengthening until they reach their peak density and strength when you reach the age of around 35. Most people don't have enough calcium in their diets or take any supplements, but it isn't until after the age of 35 that the natural effects of ageing, combined with the lack of nutrients and vitamins crucial to good bone health, really start to take their toll, triggering bone degeneration and weakness. Many osteoporosis sufferers don't even realize they have a bone problem until a fracture occurs.

What can you do?

If you're still in your twenties, the key piece of advice is to try and build up your bone strength as much as you can so that when your bones reach their peak density, you'll have more bone strength to fall back on as your skeleton starts to age and weaken. If you're in your thirties or forties, the chances are that your bones have passed their density peak so the best strategy is to try to maintain their strength for as long as possible. If you're in your fifties, you need to make sure you try everything you can to slow down the rate at which your bones are ageing, especially if you're a woman. Whatever your age, bear in mind the tips outlined on page 147.

Alzheimer's disease – what is it?

This debilitating disease is a complex form of dementia in which many types of brain degeneration take place including brain cells and the connections between them dying off, as well as damaging deposits forming in the brain. As you age, your risk of developing the disease increases – as many as 25 per cent of people over the age of 85 probably have symptoms of some form of dementia, while half a million people in the UK are known to suffer from Alzheimer's. Once the disease has been medically diagnosed, most patients live a further four to 20 years but suffer substantially increasing memory loss, language difficulties and confusion over the course of the disease.

What causes it?

While researchers have made good headway in understanding how the disease progresses, it's still not clear what factors cause it. However, there may be a genetic component – if one of your close relatives has been diagnosed with the disease, your own chances of developing it are increased.

Right: Keeping your mind active as you get older will help protect you against Alzheimer's disease.

Top tips for protecting against Alzheimer's disease

- **Eat the right fats.** Those risky animal fats, known as saturated fats, as well as artificially made fats, such as hydrogenated and trans fats, don't do your brain much good. Cut down on fatty meats, butter, margarine and processed foods and switch instead to using small amounts of healthier fats in the form of monounsaturated varieties, such as olive oil.

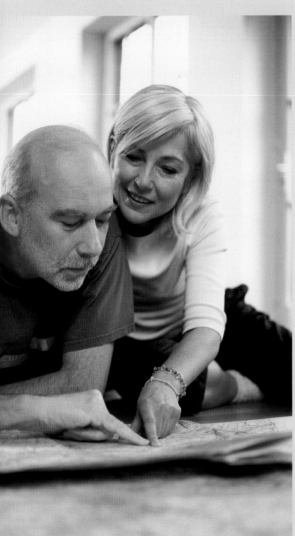

- **Eat oily fish.** Once again, the omega-3 oils found in some fish appear to boost the health of your blood vessels, heart and brain. Try eating about 100 g (3½ oz) of oily fish, for example fresh tuna, trout, anchovies, sardines, pilchards, kippers or herring, at least twice a week, or you could try taking a daily fish oil or cod liver oil supplement.

- **Don't skimp on fruit and vegetables.** They contain important vitamins, minerals and other nutrients that will keep your brain healthy (and as we've seen earlier, five portions a day will boost your overall health too). In particular, vitamin B12 and folic acid seem to have an important role in healthy cell function and help to keep levels of that potentially dangerous natural substance homocysteine down to safe levels. High levels of homocysteine have been found both in people suffering from heart disease and those with dementia, and it's likely that heart disease increases your risk of some forms of dementia, so overall, keeping homocysteine levels down is important. You should particularly try to eat lots of leafy green vegetables, such as spinach, broccoli or cabbage and, if you're over the age of 50, consider taking a vitamin B12 supplement – around 2.5 mg a day should help.

- **Keep active.** Both physical and mental activity seem to improve your chances of staying healthy for longer as you age. Stick to a regular physical exercise plan and keep your brain stimulated with regular reading, puzzles, games or even mental arithmetic.

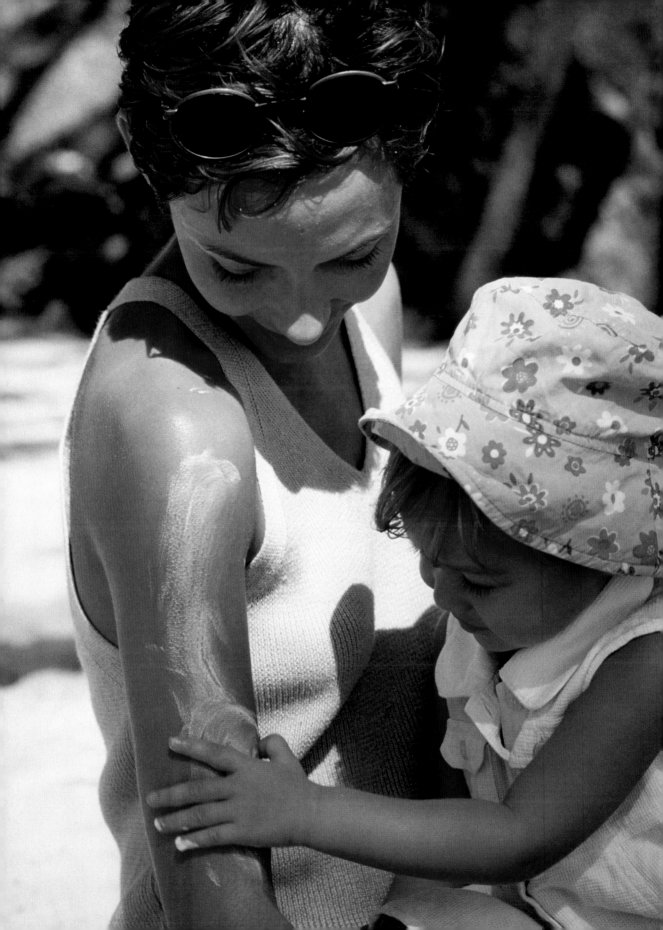

8

Ten Top Tips for Living Well

While most of us would like to stick to a long-term healthy routine, there are often times in our lives when the responsibilities of work, home and family overtake all the good health intentions. If you're tired, stressed, upset or anxious, healthy habits can be the first thing to suffer as your overall wellbeing gets pushed to the bottom of the priority list.

For many of us, this kind of day-to-day existence can end up being a way of life and, as a result, health problems can creep up unannounced. With this in mind, we've compiled our top ten tips for keeping your overall wellbeing under control – even when the going gets tough. If you can stick to these, you'll have the foundations for building long-term good health for yourself. And when life allows you some more time and energy, try out some of the extra tips we've given you in the preceding chapters.

When it comes to the tips in this chapter, as well as all the other pointers we've suggested along the way, always remember three key rules. First, when you're thinking about any lifestyle change, work out a realistic goal, otherwise you'll simply be setting yourself up for failure. Exercising every day could indeed improve your health, but you may find you simply do not have the time, so if you try it and can't stick to it, you're going to end up feeling discouraged and negative about yourself. Second, when you try a wellbeing tip, give the change a chance. Some people simply flit between one piece of advice and another, always seeking out a new solution to their health concern, but you need to give these things time to work. Finally, reward yourself for taking the time and making the effort to change your ways – feeling good about yourself will enhance your wellbeing even further.

Top tip 1

Have at least two or three alcohol-free days a week

Drinking alcohol in moderation is an enjoyable and relaxing part of social life, but it's all too easy to suffer poor health if you start drinking too much. Think carefully about how much you drink each week and remember that the recommended maximum amount of alcohol is 28 units per week for men and 21 units per week for women (refer to pages 21–31 if you need more information on this). Essentially, this amounts to three to four standard alcoholic drinks per day for men and two to three per day for women, but remember that these figures are a maximum guideline on alcohol consumption. In our opinion, having at least two or three alcohol-free days a week will give your body a chance to recover and recharge. This doesn't mean that you can binge on alcohol on the remaining days of the week, but by having alcohol-free days you should lower your overall dependence, which means you should drink less alcohol on other days too – giving you a healthier body (and bank balance!).

How to do it

● At the start of each week, decide in advance which are going to be your alcohol-free days. The start of the week might be easier as social events tend to occur nearer the weekend.

● Find an alternative non-alcoholic drink you enjoy. If water on its own doesn't satisfy you, try flavouring it with a slice of lemon or lime or have a soda, mineral water or tonic water (although it's better to pick a diet or low-calorie one as the other types can be high in sugar).

● It's very important to drink plenty of water every day – most of us walk around in a mild state of dehydration – and remember that because alcohol is a diuretic (it makes you urinate more liquid than you've taken in by drinking), it's vital that you drink even more water on days when you're consuming alcohol. You should be drinking at least eight tall glasses of water a day and even more if you regularly drink coffee or caffeinated soft drinks.

● Rather than occasionally managing a tiny plastic cup of water from your workplace water cooler, if you have one, buy a 2-litre (3½-pint) bottle of mineral water and fill it up from the water cooler at the start of each day – that way, you know exactly how much you're getting through and whether or not you need to drink more.

● While suddenly increasing the amount of water you drink will mean more frequent trips to the bathroom at first, don't despair as your kidneys will adjust in a day or two and you won't feel the need to urinate as often.

● When it does come to drinking alcohol, try to drink a glass of water for every alcoholic drink you have. This should limit the short-term problematic effects of alcohol (and the chances of you being hungover the next day), but it also reduces your chances of binge-drinking too.

Remember: It's not just alcoholics who experience liver damage and disease, cancers of the mouth and throat, brain damage, diabetes, heart problems and ulcers as a result of drinking alcohol. Unless you drink moderately, your risk of all of the above will be substantially increased.

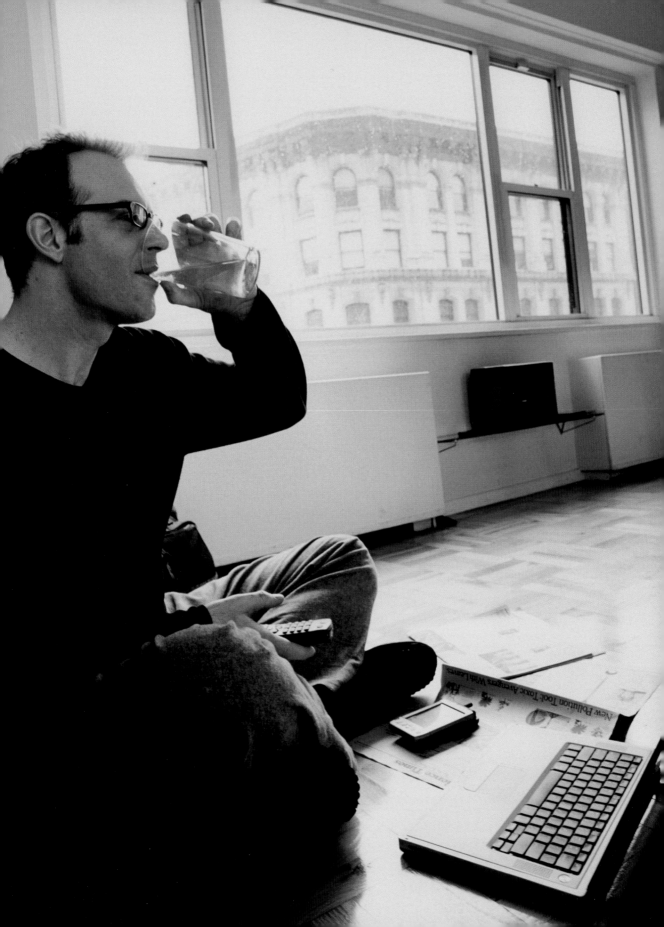

Top tip 2

Quit smoking. If you're a non-smoker, limit the amount of time you spend in smoky environments

Whether you enjoy smoking, plan to give it up one day soon or are desperately trying to give up right now, the message is simple. Cigarettes significantly harm your health and cause five million people around the world to die prematurely every year. If you're a smoker, your cigarette habit should be the first lifestyle change you tackle. If you're a non-smoker, your long-term health will be improved by trying to avoid smoky environments altogether or at least cutting down the amount of time you spend in them. We're not pretending that giving up smoking is easy – nicotine's a highly addictive drug, which explains why a staggering 570 billion cigarettes get smoked around the world every year (80 billion of those by smokers in the UK), but the health benefits are more than worth the effort of giving up.

How to do it

● There are many ways you can try to kick the habit, so first choose one that appeals to you most: you might want to try going 'cold turkey', joining a local support group or using nicotine-replacement treatments, such as gum or patches (the latter have been shown to double your chances of successfully giving up).

● Whatever your choice, pick a date in your diary when you're going to start being a non-smoker – and stick to it.

● Throw out all your smoking paraphernalia – physical triggers, such as lighters, ashtrays and matches could tip you into having a cigarette when you're going through withdrawal.

● Tell your friends and family about your plan. If any of them are smokers, you might need to give them a wide berth for a while. Lean on the non-smokers you know for support and encouragement.

● Avoid places and situations where others will be smoking – for the first few weeks at least. Accept that you are going to be tempted to have another cigarette so it's best to minimize the possible social triggers.

● If you feel low or irritable, do some physical exercise: try running, swimming or a bike ride. You'll soon be enjoying better physical fitness and stamina as a result of giving up smoking – and, in the meantime, having a workout will improve your mood and energy levels.

● Try not to over-eat to compensate for the lack of cigarettes. Stock up on healthy food, such as fresh fruit, nuts, raisins and chopped carrots, which you can snack on whenever you feel tempted to have a cigarette.

● Buy yourself a present or treat with the money you've saved by giving up.

● If you're struggling, ask for help. You could try your doctor, a pharmacist or a local support group or telephone helpline.

Remember: It's estimated that one in two long-term smokers will end up dying prematurely as a result of their habit – and half of those will die in their middle age.

Top tip 3

Reduce your intake of bad fats

Healthy eating doesn't have to be boring or unpleasurable. By following the three simple changes in top tips 3, 4 and 5, you'll find that your diet will be instantly more nutritious and beneficial, without leaving you feeling dissatisfied. While we all know that high-fat diets can result in weight gain and poor health, your body does need some fat to function properly, as we saw in Chapter 1 (see page 13). Some of the most important vitamins you get from your food (A, D and E) are fat soluble – for that reason alone, it's important not to go too low-fat and don't even consider no-fat. Not all fats are bad for you, so if you can learn which ones to stop eating and which ones to replace them with, you'll be well on track for good, long-term nutrition and health, while also still being able to enjoy tasty and satisfying food.

How to do it

● Saturated fats are the baddies – you'll find those in meat (especially red meat) and full-fat dairy products, such as cream, butter and cheese. These will all increase your levels of LDL (low-density lipoprotein) cholesterol, which is dangerous for your heart.

● Because saturated fats tend to be cheaper, you'll also find that most processed and pre-prepared foods contain them or other baddies like hydrogenated or trans fats.

● Switch to low-fat milk and use fromage frais or low-fat yoghurt instead of cream.

● For cooking, use monounsaturated fats, such as olive oil or, for a less expensive option, try polyunsaturated ones like sunflower oil. Both these still contain the same amount of calories as saturated fats, so you need to use them only in small amounts, but they're far better for your heart's health as they don't have the same effect on your LDL levels and may even increase levels of the good protective cholesterol, HDL (high-density lipoprotein).

● If you're eating bread with dinner, try dipping it in a small amount of olive oil instead of spreading on butter – add a dash of balsamic vinegar to make it all the more delicious. For breakfast toast or lunchtime sandwiches, use an olive-oil-based spread. Although margarine is made from a polyunsaturated form of fat, some are chemically altered to make the product last longer. This turns the fat into what's known as a trans fat, and nutritionists believe that this is even worse for your health than saturated fat. Stick to monounsaturated types of fat, such as olive oil. If in any doubt, check the label. If it mentions anything about 'hydrogenated vegetable oil' or 'hydrogenated fat', that means it has been processed and is now a trans fat, so steer clear.

● Remember that adding fat to food is the cheapest and easiest way to add flavour, so restaurant food tends to be laden with the worst kind of saturated fats. When you're eating out, try to pick food that's been grilled or baked. Avoid ordering menu options that have been been fried or are served with buttery or cream-based sauces.

Remember: Research has shown that even a two per cent cut in your intake of the worst kind of processed saturated fats could reduce the risk of coronary heart disease by up to a quarter.

Top tip 4

Eat at least five portions of fruit and vegetables every day

By including more fruit and vegetables in your daily diet, you can drastically reduce your chances of developing a number of major diseases. In fact, a recent study showed that with each extra portion a day, you lower your risk of heart disease by four per cent and your risk of a stroke by six per cent. Eating lots of fruit and vegetables also substantially reduces your risk of developing cancer, especially cancers of the colon, stomach and breast. What's more, fruit and vegetables are packed with energy and nutrients that will improve your body's everyday functioning. In the UK, the majority of us eat only three of the recommended portions a day, so getting the maximum benefits should only involve a small, inexpensive and easy increase for most people.

How to do it
- One portion of fruit equals half a large fruit, such as a melon or grapefruit, or two small fruits, for example apples or satsumas.

- A handful of dried fruit, for instance raisins or dried apricots, also counts as one portion.

- A single glass of pure fruit juice counts as a portion, but it can only count as one no matter how much you drink as juice contains far less fibre than other fruits and vegetables.

- One portion of vegetables equals three tablespoonfuls of raw or cooked vegetables – fresh, tinned or frozen all count.

- A small bowl of salad counts as one portion of vegetables.

- Pulses and beans count as one portion, but like the fruit juice they can only count as one, no matter how much you eat, because they don't contain as many nutrients as other vegetable options (although they are very rich in fibre).

- To get the maximum benefit in terms of nutrients and protection against diseases, you need to eat a mix of different fruit and vegetables to make up your five portions every day.

- If you find it hard to notch up the full five portions a day, try putting a fruit bowl out on your desk at work, in a prominent place in your kitchen or on a dining or coffee table. Research shows you're far more likely to eat fruit if it's visible rather than being hidden away inside your fridge.

- Have a portion of fruit or vegetables for your morning or afternoon snack, instead of biscuits, sweets or crisps. Try a large banana or a handful of chopped carrots.

Remember: If you eat at least five portions of fruit and vegetables every day, you'll be cutting your risk of heart disease, stroke and cancer by as much as 20 per cent.

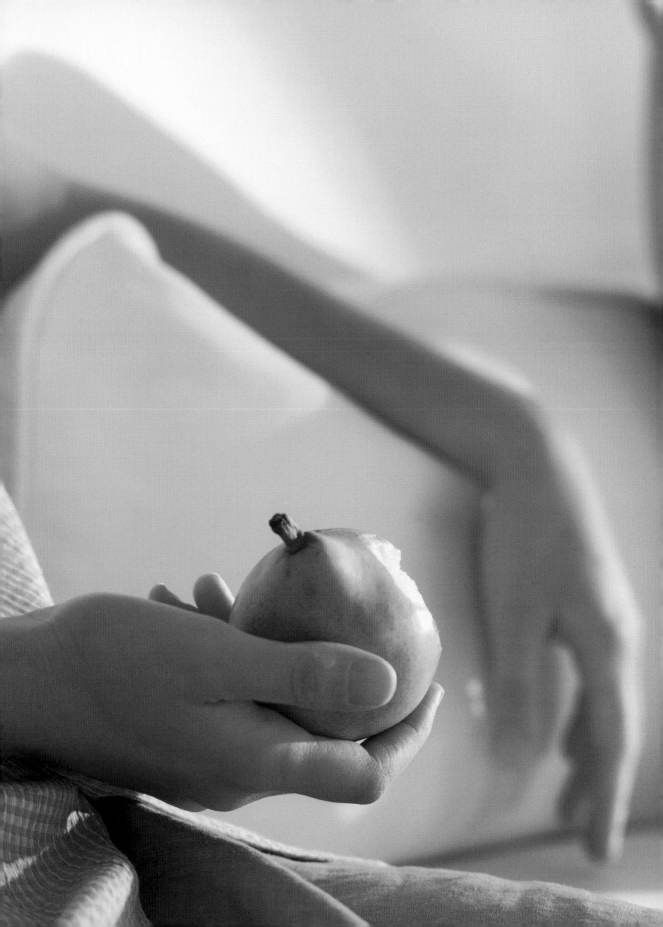

Top tip 5

Cut down on sugars

We don't just mean stop eating sweets and chocolate, we're also talking about curbing carbohydrates generally. Carbohydrates (sugars) do offer a quick supply of energy, but remember that they're also responsible for your body releasing the hormone insulin, which turns excess sugars into fat and is responsible for storing fat too. If you eat food containing a very high amount of carbohydrate, there'll be a sudden rise in your blood sugar level. Aside from the fact that, unless you happen to be exercising vigorously, most of this will simply get stored as fat, spiking your blood sugar in this way tends to tip your body into an emergency balancing mode so that in just a short period of time, you'll hit a blood sugar low that will trigger further carbohydrate cravings, tiredness and irritability.

How to do it

● If you need further convincing of how high-carbohydrate foods affect your energy levels, try the following test. Next time you hit a four-in-the-afternoon energy low, eat a chocolate bar. It's almost guaranteed that within about an hour, you'll be craving something more to eat because of that blood sugar spike. The next day, try eating a low-sugar snack, such as an apple or better still, a protein-rich one like a few slices of low-fat cheese or a handful of nuts. You'll get slower-burning energy that lasts for longer and shouldn't trigger the same carbohydrate cravings later on.

● Remember that all refined, processed carbohydrates, such as white bread, rice and pasta are very high in sugar. Try switching to wholemeal bread, brown rice and wholewheat pasta. You don't have to give up your favourite foods, just try to adapt them to limit your sugar intake. Wholegrain foods still contain sugars, but they're of a type that your body takes much longer to break down so they won't cause your blood sugar to fluctuate as severely and are less likely to get stored as fat.

● Don't deny yourself the occasional high-carbohydrate treat. But do try to limit these to the morning or early afternoon, when you're going to be most active and more likely to use up the sugars you're consuming. In the evening as you relax and unwind, then head off to bed, high-carbohydrate foods are far more likely to end up as stored fat.

● As well as limiting your intake of sugary food such as sweets and biscuits, watch out for hidden sugars in foods that you might think are healthy and nutritious. Many breakfast cereals are loaded with added sugar. And check out a few labels for the carbohydrate levels of even the purest fruit juices (that claim 'no added sugar'): the juicing process tends to push the natural sugars out of the fruit's cells, so if you drink several glasses of fruit juice a day, you'll be consuming a lot of extra sugar. For example, an average-sized orange contains around 14 g of carbohydrate (natural fruit sugars), while a single serving of orange juice contains as much as 26 g. If you're a fruit juice fan, try drinking it diluted half and half with water.

Remember: Added sugars offer no nutritional value, just 'empty calories'. A standard can of cola contains a staggering seven teaspoons of sugar – so cutting back on foods containing added sugar is a big step towards controlling energy levels, cravings and weight gain.

Top tip 6

Protect yourself from the sun

Since bronzed bodies were first linked with glamour in the 1920s, we've exposed ourselves to ever-increasing amounts of the sun's rays. The advent of cheap package holidays and budget air travel in recent years has made hot exotic countries far more accessible. Nowadays, most of us think of two weeks spent basking in foreign sunshine as the very epitomy of rest and relaxation, but as we saw in more detail in Chapter 4 (see pages 83–5), the sun's potentially harmful UV rays can end up causing serious damage when it comes to your health. Protecting yourself from the sun doesn't mean you can't still enjoy a summer holiday abroad or leisure time spent outdoors – you just need to make some simple lifestyle changes in order to minimize the harmful effects of UV exposure to your skin.

How to do it

● Don't rely on sun protection (listed in ingredients as SPF) added to moisturizers or make-up as you're unlikely to apply enough of the product to make any real difference to your skin in terms of UV protection. Instead, invest in a good oil-free face protection cream with at least SPF 15 and apply it to your face each morning, whether or not it's the height of summer.

● Once you are on that summer holiday, you should be using creams with an SPF of at least 25. Make sure you apply them to all areas of exposed skin at least 30 minutes before you go in the sun, so that you get the cream's full protective effect.

● Don't skimp on the amount of cream you apply – in terms of protecting your skin from UV, the more cream you put on and the more frequently you apply it, the better.

● Wear a sun hat and sunglasses, and cover up as much of your skin as you can.

● Sit in the shade and especially avoid going out in the sun during the hottest hours of the day – between 11 a.m. and 3 p.m.

● If you're desperate to be bronzed, use fake tan products rather than sun beds or lying out in the sun. But don't forget that fake tans don't offer UV protection, so you still need to use those sun creams to protect yourself.

● If you do go out in the sun, avoid getting sunburnt at all costs. A nasty case of sunburn can double your chances of developing skin cancer.

Remember: A natural tan won't develop until the sun's UV rays have already begun to cause damage inside your skin's cells – and the results of that damage start with premature ageing and end in skin cancer.

Top tip 7

Be physically active

As we've mentioned throughout this book, taking regular exercise is a great all-round means of improving your health and wellbeing. It reduces your risk of dying prematurely from heart disease and many forms of cancer, and helps control your weight, blood pressure and the health of your bones, joints and muscles. What's more, it has been proven to boost your mood and fight depression, anxiety and stress. While keeping fit at the gym or taking part in sports is the best way to get the health benefits of exercise, there are plenty of other ways to keep physically active if you're short of time.

How to do it

- If you take part in sports or have a gym routine, exercising for 30 minutes three times a week should be fine, otherwise try to incorporate physical activity into your daily life as often as you can.

- Remember you need to get your heart rate up to get the maximum benefit from exercise. If you're relying on everyday physical activity, such as walking briskly, going up and down stairs or even cleaning the house, you'll need to be working hard enough that you get slightly breathless to be sure that your heart is getting a decent workout.

- While you don't need to exercise strenuously to get the basic health rewards, research shows that the benefits can be increased by exercising more intensively, more frequently and for longer periods of time. But remember that it's also possible

to overdo it – refer back to Chapter 3 (see pages 58–61) for more information on exercise addiction.

- You don't have to complete 30 minutes of physical activity in a single block to get the benefit. Research has shown that three blocks of 10 minutes or two blocks of 15 minutes of activity are just as effective.

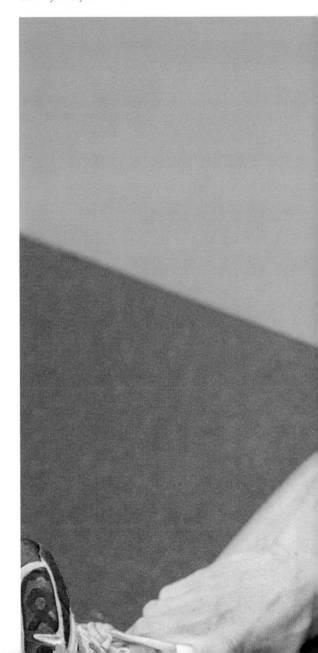

● It's well worth consulting a doctor or a professional trainer before you embark on a new regular exercise programme.

● Always take a rest from exercise if you experience pain, or if you've got an injury or you're unwell.

Remember: There is not one other single lifestyle choice – or indeed, medical intervention – that can offer the vast health benefits that regular exercise can in terms of reducing your risks of illness, disease and premature death.

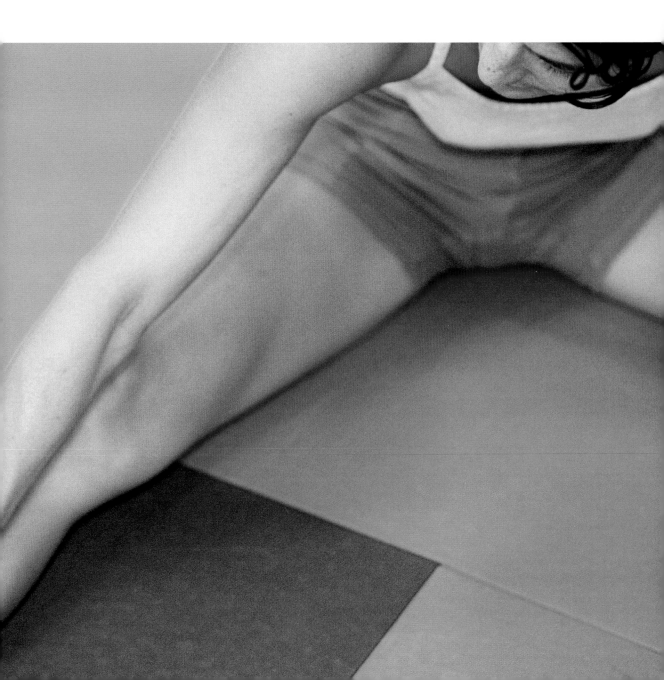

Top tip 8

Keep a close eye on your health

In the rush of everyday life, most of us tend not to think too much about major health problems, especially if everything's in working order. However, the fact remains that almost all illnesses and diseases can be tackled and treated much more effectively if they're diagnosed early, as we saw in Chapter 7. Keeping a regular eye on your health is a good habit to get into, whatever your age or family health history. Follow our guidelines below for what you can check yourself and what you should have checked by a medical professional. While worrying obsessively about your health is clearly a problem in itself, if you can stick to our suggestions on how often you need to check yourself, you should get all the benefits while also limiting any health anxieties.

How to do it

- If you're a woman, you should check your breasts, nipples and armpits for any unusual changes, swellings or lumps once a month. Just after your period is a good time to do this, after the swelling and discomfort in your breasts caused by pre-menstrual hormonal changes has settled down.

- If you're a man, you should check your testicles for any unusual changes, swellings, soreness or lumps every month or so.

- Everyone should inspect their skin monthly, paying particular attention to all your moles or large freckles to see whether they've changed size, shape, colour or texture. Ask a partner or friend to check moles that are on your back.

- Everyone should keep an eye on their bowel movements and check for any unusual symptoms, such as traces of blood or mucus, or any other unexpected changes in their bowel habits.

- Every couple of months, have a good look inside your mouth at your teeth, gums and tongue. Look out for any bleeding from your gums, or gums that seem to have receded along the gum-line. Check also for any ulcers, swellings or sore spots that don't seem to be healing properly. If you find any of these, visit your dentist for a check-up.

- You should be attending a regular check-up with a dentist at least once a year.

- It's important to have your eyes tested by an optometrist at least once every two years. You will need to be checked more often if you wear glasses or contact lenses.

- If you think that unless you're experiencing any symptoms, eye and teeth check-ups are unnecessary and a waste of time and money, think again. You only have one pair of eyes and one set of teeth and once they're gone, your quality of life is going to be drastically affected. What's more, regular checks at the dentist and optometrist can also reveal underlying serious conditions, such as high blood pressure, diabetes, and brain and mouth tumours.

- If you experience a significant period of stress, it's worth going to the doctor to have your blood pressure checked.

- If you're a woman and you experience menstrual problems, such as very heavy or

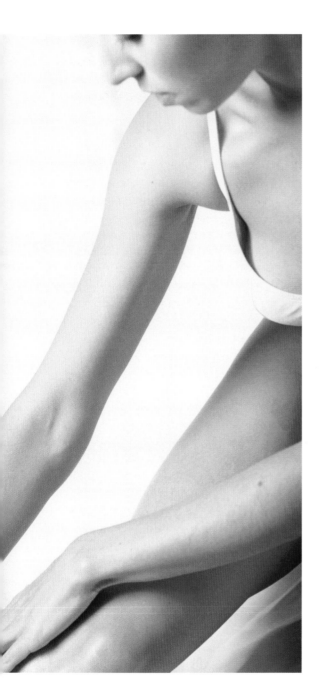

- It's extremely important to make sure you attend regular cervical smears (or pap tests) if you're a sexually active woman aged between 21 and 64 and also mammograms (breast x-rays) if your doctor asks you to have one (it's usually only women over 50 who are called for regular mammograms, unless you've consulted your doctor about an unusual breast symptom or you have a genetic predisposition to breast cancer).

- If you're sexually active, it's worth having a sexual check-up once a year. Even if you're in a monogamous, long-term relationship, problems can still occur due to bacterial and yeast infections.

- If you're over 40, it might be worth asking your doctor about having an annual medical check-up to test your cholesterol levels, blood pressure and for other conditions that are more likely to affect you as you age.

- If you experience any persistent unusual symptoms in any part of your body or are worried about any ongoing aspect of your health, do see a doctor. Don't soldier on self-medicating with over-the-counter treatments if they're making no difference. Likewise, don't rely on medical information you find on the Internet and in magazines. The best solution is always to consult a doctor about health problems.

Remember: No matter how well you feel, being body-aware is one of your key weapons in the fight against poor health, illness and disease. In almost all cases, early detection will drastically improve your chances of successful treatment, recovery and survival.

irregular periods, or any gynaecological discomfort or pain, it's very important that you see your doctor or a specialist. Don't suffer in silence.

Top tip 9

Have better sex – and more of it

When you're stressed or tired, your sex life can be the first thing to suffer. But scientific research has shown that there are substantial health benefits to be had by having regular sex – assuming, that is, that you are protecting yourself properly from sexually transmitted infections (for more information on STIs, refer to pages 128–31). In a ten-year study of nearly 1000 middle-aged men in Wales, researchers discovered that the men who reported having orgasms most frequently had less than half the risk of dying prematurely as the other men, especially from coronary heart disease. Other studies have reported that even having sex just twice a week seems to offer a boost to your immune system and hormone levels. Most importantly, sex is a great form of exercise, which means improved circulation, blood pressure and lower LDL cholesterol levels.

How to do it

● If you're single, don't despair. Use this opportunity to explore your own sexuality in more depth and work out what you'd like to experience sexually in your next relationship.

● If you're in a relationship, you and your partner need to make time for sex. Schedule in some early nights or a lie-in at the weekend. Remember, the more frequently you have sex, the higher your hormone levels will be, so you'll both have greater sexual appetites.

● If you've got young children, consider fitting a lock on your bedroom door so you can have sex without fear of an unexpected intrusion at an inappropriate moment. Or ask your parents, in-laws or family friends to have the kids to stay for a weekend, to allow you and your partner the time and space to concentrate on boosting your sex life and your relationship.

● If you're concerned that you and your partner have differing sex drives, likes or dislikes, try to talk openly about this with him or her. Don't save concerns up for when you get down to it in the bedroom, but instead discuss any issues at a time when you're both calm, refreshed and sober.

● Don't get stuck in a sexual rut. Human beings are creatures of habit but, after a while, this can take the pleasure out of sex. Make the effort to keep things fresh and exciting by exploring and experimenting with new techniques, positions and locations.

● Anxieties about contraception or concerns about trying to get pregnant can both stop sex being enjoyable. It's worth discussing any issues with your doctor or a counsellor so that minor problems don't snowball into major relationship issues.

● To experience better sex, try some Kegel or pelvic-floor exercises. Next time you urinate, try stopping the urine in mid-flow. The muscles you use to do this are your pelvic-floor muscles. By tensing these several times for five minutes twice a day, you will improve sexual sensations and the intensity of your orgasms.

Remember: Thirty minutes of active sex burns up the same number of calories as running on a treadmill for 15 minutes – about 200. Regular sex gives you and your partner the health benefits of exercise and does wonders for the emotional health of your relationship too.

Top tip 10

Enjoy your body

Most of us spend far too long worrying about looks, shapes and sizes when it comes to our bodies. In our culture, that's perfectly understandable, but the fact is that this kind of negativity feeds a vicious circle of anxiety, low confidence and guilt. It's well worth trying to shift the focus of your feelings about your body towards what a miracle it really is. What's more, if you can keep your body healthy and in peak condition, you'll be able to enjoy even more of its incredible abilities. Think of exercise as a way of experiencing and enjoying your body's extraordinary physical capacities, while eating healthily is a means of feeding your body what it needs to pump you full of energy and strength. If you respect your body and treat it well, it will serve you better and for longer.

How to do it

● Try to connect with your body more regularly. Most of us have desk-bound jobs and spend all day using our brains rather than our bodies. Use exercise, everyday physical activity or even social events like dancing to reconnect with your body. If you pay more attention to it and learn how to tune into the messages it sends your brain, you'll find you'll be more in touch with it when you really are hungry, full, tired or in pain.

● Be in control of your body, don't let it control you. Knowing exactly what certain types of foods do to your body or precisely how exercise can help your health will spur you on to fight cravings, maintain a healthy weight and steer clear of bad habits. Ignorance certainly isn't bliss when it comes

to your health, so be informed and use that knowledge to be healthy and stay that way.

● Don't let keeping your body healthy become an obsession. The occasional treat keeps life interesting and varied, and stops you feeling like you're denying yourself what you fancy now and again. You can savour and enjoy the pleasures of life while still being healthy – and staying that way.

Remember: True wellbeing is when health, pleasure and happiness blend together. Eat well, stay fit, feel good about yourself and enjoy the best of what life has to offer. Here's to your good health!

Useful Information

If you would like further information on anything we've covered in this book, we recommend you contact the following organizations or look at the listed websites.

General health

World Health Organization
www.who.int/
Tel: +41 22 791 2111 (headquarters)
International authority on research into all aspects of health around the globe. The website gives a fascinating and comprehensive insight into worldwide health issues.

English Department of Health
www.doh.gov.uk
Tel: 020 7210 4850 (customer service centre)
The official website of the government's Department of Health offers extensive information and guidelines for a number of major health topics.

Patient UK
www.patient.org.uk/
Tel: 0113 259 1122 (general enquiries)
This invaluable website offers leaflets on a myriad health topics, links to other sources of information on the web and contact information for many support groups and organizations.

British Association of Counsellors and Psychotherapists
www.bacp.co.uk/
Tel: 0870 443 5252
Look in the Public Information section on the website for explanations of what to expect from therapy. This site also offers a useful search engine that locates fully registered therapists in your local area.

British Association of Behavioural and Cognitive Psychotherapies
www.babcp.org.uk/
Tel: 01254 875277
It's also worth contacting this association for useful information on therapy and finding a therapist.

Healthy eating & nutrition

Food Standards Agency
www.food.gov.uk/
Tel: 020 7276 8000
An excellent, comprehensive website aimed specifically at consumers, packed with information on nutrition, healthy eating and the truth about food scares.

British Dietetic Association
www.bda.uk.com/
Tel: 0121 200 8080
Useful association through which you can find a registered dietitian in your local area for personal advice on nutrition.

British Nutrition Foundation
www.nutrition.org.uk/
Tel: 020 7404 6504
Information-packed website with easy-to-digest factsheets and leaflets on many aspects of healthy eating, for all ages.

Medical Research Council Human Nutrition Research
www.mrc-hnr.cam.ac.uk
Tel: 01223 426356
Reviews a wide range of academic and scientific research studies on many aspects of nutrition.

The Nutrition Society
www.nutritionsociety.org.uk/
Tel: 020 7371 6225
This is the largest scientific group studying nutrition in Europe. Their website provides details of scientific studies and research at the academic end of the nutrition field.

Drinking

Institute of Alcohol Studies
www.ias.org.uk/
Tel: 020 7222 4001
The Institute's website contains excellent factsheets and papers with straightforward information and advice on sensible drinking.

Health Promotion England – Think About Drink
www.wrecked.co.uk
Tel: 020 7210 4850 (general number for NHS)
This NHS website is aimed at young people and is designed to give all sorts of information on the effects of alcohol in a very accessible style.

Alcohol Concern
www.alcoholconcern.org.uk/
Tel: 020 7928 7377
The UK's national agency on alcohol misuse. The website has lots of information and factsheets about problem drinking and how to get help for yourself or someone else.

Alcoholics Anonymous
www.alcoholics-anonymous.org.uk/
Tel: 01904 644026
The easy-to-use website directs you to self-help groups and meetings in your local area and offers a confidential and anonymous telephone service for advice and support.

Al-Anon UK & Eire
www.al-anonuk.org.uk/
Tel: 0141 339 8884 (24-hour helpline) or
020 7403 0888 (general enquiries)
This excellent site is specifically designed to offer help and support to the friends and family of those with drinking problems.

Drugs

Drugscope
www.drugscope.org.uk/
Tel: 020 7928 1211
The UK's leading advisory centre on drug use. Their informative website offers clear, accessible information on all aspects of drug-taking and a directory of drug treatment services where you can find help and advice locally.

Talk to Frank
www.talktofrank.com/
Tel: 0800 776600
Building on the work of the original National Drugs Helpline, this excellent website offers comprehensive information, advice and support for anyone concerned about drugs, and a free confidential 24-hour helpline.

Drugworld
www.drugworld.org/
Tel: 020 7702 2300 (Turning Point head office)
A website put together by the charity Turning Point, designed to give young people the straight-talking low-down on drugs.

Narcotics Anonymous
www.ukna.org/
Tel: 020 7730 0009
The UK arm of the international organization that offers help, advice and a network of support groups in local areas.

Exercise & fitness

BBC Health's fitness section
www.bbc.co.uk/health/fitness/
Comprehensive information on all aspects of exercise from the BBC's health website, for all ages and activity levels.

NHS Direct
www.nhsdirect.nhs.uk/
Tel: 0845 4647 (nurse advice)
The exercise section on this health website run by the NHS offers good advice on incorporating more activity into your daily life, especially for those new to exercise.

Exercise Register
www.exerciseregister.com/
Tel: 020 8325 1328
This useful website offers a directory of health clubs, leisure centres, gyms, qualified personal trainers and exercise consultants in all areas.

Stress, anxiety & depression

Mind

www.mind.org.uk/

Tel: 0845 766 0163

The UK mental health charity's website offers a wide range of information and advice on how to get support and treatment for mental health issues.

Sane

www.sane.org.uk/

Tel: 0845 767 8000

Another mental health charity whose website provides very clear and accessible information, resources and support. They also offer a confidential national helpline number.

Anxiety Care

www.anxietycare.org.uk/

Tel: 020 8262 8891 or 020 8262 8892

This charity specializes in helping people recover from anxiety disorders. They offer free advice and support from trained counsellors, a chatroom and lots of information.

Depression Alliance

www.depressionalliance.org/

Tel: 0845 123 2320

The leading UK charity supporting people with depression. Their website gives plenty of clear information about the condition, its treatment, support and advice.

The Samaritans

www.samaritans.org/

Tel: 08457 909090

The Samaritans offer a 24-hour confidential emotional support telephone line for anyone suffering from worry, distress, despair or even suicidal feelings. Their website gives useful answers to frequently asked questions about calling and plenty of other information.

Sleep

National Sleep Foundation (USA)

www.sleepfoundation.org/

Tel: +1 202 347 3471

A very accessible and useful website that gives thorough explanations on all aspects of sleep.

Sleep Education

www.sleepeducation.com/

Tel: +1 708 492 0930

An interesting and easy-to-use American website that offers lots of information on sleep, sleep disorders and links to other resources.

Loughborough Sleep Research Centre

www.lboro.ac.uk/departments/hu/groups/sleep/

Tel: 01509 223091

The UK's world-renowned sleep research centre. Their fascinating website offers clear explanations on sleep research projects, interesting articles and advice.

Travel health

MASTA

www.masta.org/

Tel: 0113 238 7575

UK organization dedicated to providing up-to-date information on travel health with information on specific destinations and particular focus on vaccinations and anti-malarial medication.

English Department of Health

www.dh.gov.uk/PolicyAndGuidance/HealthAdvice ToTravellers

Tel: 020 7210 4850 (customer service centre)

This government website gives lots of helpful advice about travel health and explains how to get reciprocal health treatment (on the NHS) with an E111 form in the European Union and some non-EU countries.

Flight Health

www.flighthealth.org/

A very useful independent on-line resource packed with information on a wide range of health issues associated with jet travel, such as DVT and jet lag.

The Skin Cancer Foundation

www.skincancer.org/

Tel: +1 212 725 5751

The website of this American foundation gives extremely clear information on preventing sun damage and skin cancer, with excellent advice on how to examine your skin for any symptoms.

Acne

Acne Support Group

www.m2w3.com/acne/

Tel: 0870 870 2263

A clear and concise website with lots of facts and frequently asked questions about acne.

Stop Spots

www.stopspots.org/

Tel: 0870 870 2263

The Acne Support Group's alternative website designed specifically for teenagers. Excellently written and ideal for any young person experiencing acne.

Acne Net

www.skincarephysicians.com/acnenet/

Tel: +1 847 330 0230

The American Academy of Dermatology runs this informative and accessible website explaining acne.

Sweating

Hyperhidrosis Support Group

www.hyperhidrosisuk.org/

A helpful UK website aimed at people who suffer from excessive sweating.

Hairloss

Hairloss Talk

www.hairlosstalk.com/

Tel: +1 619 280 4994

An excellent independent American website that discusses hair loss, its treatments and offers comprehensive resources and a discussion forum for support and advice.

Embarrassing Problems

www.embarrassingproblems.com/

Tel: 01235 523233

An interesting and practical website on the type of health problems you might not find easy to discuss. Search for the clear and information-packed section on hair loss, how it happens and what you can do about it.

Body image

Eating Disorders Association

www.edauk.com/

Tel: 0870 770 3256

The first port-of-call for information and advice on all types of eating disorders. The website also offers access to support groups and treatment services.

About Face

www.about-face.org/

Tel: +1 415 436 0212

This interesting and positive American website looks at the roots of distorted feelings about body image in women.

Body Positive

www.bodypositive.com/

Tel: +1 650 321 2606

This American website is packed with articles, information, advice and tips on how to boost your body image.

British Association of Aesthetic Plastic Surgery

www.baaps.org.uk/

Tel: 020 7405 2234

If you're determined to go under the knife, make sure you know your facts and use this association to find a reputable and properly qualified plastic surgeon.

Attraction & love

BBC Science

www.bbc.co.uk/science/hottopics/love/

Interesting information on the science of attraction and love.

Fertility

Getting Pregnant

www.gettingpregnant.co.uk/

An excellent first port-of-call website packed with all manner of information about conceiving a baby.

Human Fertilisation and Embryology Authority

www.hfea.gov.uk/

Tel: 020 7377 5077

The UK government department that regulates and licences all fertility treatment centres. Their website offers useful information and guides, plus a clinic-finding option.

Infertility Network UK

www.child.org.uk/

Tel: 01424 732 361

A very useful website with clear, easy-to-understand fact sheets written by experts in the field of reproductive medicine.

Fertility Friends

www.fertilityfriends.co.uk/

An excellent on-line resource for couples in the UK who are experiencing fertility problems. The website offers news, advice, a directory of treatment centres, local support groups and message boards.

Sexual health

Family Planning Association
www.fpa.org.uk/
Tel: 0845 310 1334 (national helpline)
The Association provides clear, concise information on sexual health, including contraception, along with details of where to get free, confidential advice and medical treatment for all sexually transmitted infections.

Herpes Viruses Association
www.herpes.org.uk/
Tel: 020 7609 9061
An ideal first port-of-call if you have any concerns or queries about herpes. The website is packed with advice and information and also offers support groups around the country.

Terrence Higgins Trust
www.tht.org.uk/
Tel: 0845 122 1200
The Trust's website is excellent for anyone wanting more information, facts or advice about HIV or AIDS. They also have a confidential telephone helpline and offer testing services across the UK.

Heart disease

BBC Health
www.bbc.co.uk/health/heart/
A clear and accessible website about all aspects of heart health. A good starting point for anyone concerned about improving the health of their heart or finding out more information on how to minimize lifestyle risks.

British Heart Foundation
www.bhf.org.uk/
Tel: 08450 708070 (heart information line)
The Foundation's extremely comprehensive website is packed with information on all aspects of how your heart works and how to keep it healthy. It also provides useful explanations of different types of heart disease and the medical treatments on offer.

Cancer

Cancer BACUP
www.cancerbacup.org.uk/
Tel: 0808 800 1234 (information line)
This organization offers a huge amount of factual and practical information, including a free telephone helpline. Their on-line resource is excellent for anyone diagnosed with cancer and their families, friends or carers, with its many links to local organizations that can offer support, help and advice.

Roy Castle Lung Cancer Foundation
www.roycastle.org/
Tel: 0871 220 5426
This charity is specifically devoted to lung cancer. Their website offers excellent information on prevention, treatment and links to local support networks.

Colon Cancer Concern
www.coloncancer.org.uk/
Tel: 08708 506050 (infoline)
This informative charity is dedicated to people with colon cancer. Their very helpful website has information on prevention, treatment and lots of links for help and advice.

Breast Cancer Care

www.breastcancercare.org.uk

Tel: 020 7384 2984

The UK's leading breast cancer charity offers information on how to be breast-aware via a telephone helpline and a useful website, which also has loads of sources of practical support and advice.

Jo's Trust

www.jotrust.co.uk/

Tel: 01327 361787

This organization is specifically for women with cervical cancer. It offers a free confidential medical helpline, and a supportive bulletin board and other sources of help and advice on its website.

Orchid Cancer Appeal

www.orchid-cancer.org.uk/

Tel: 020 7601 7808

An excellent website for anyone concerned about testicular or prostate cancers. It includes clear and straightforward details about how to examine yourself and what to look out for and there's also a forum for support and advice.

Prostate Cancer Charity

www.prostate-cancer.org.uk/

Tel: 0845 300 8383 (confidential helpline)

As well as offering a confidential helpline, this charity has a very informative and helpful website for men concerned about prostate cancer, where you'll find a 3D prostate-finder plus many other sources of information and support.

Other illness links

Action on Smoking and Health

www.ash.org.uk/

Tel: 020 7739 5902

Particularly useful for anyone trying to give up smoking, this organization has a number of telephone helplines, as well as a website with excellent tips on how to give up successfully and links to other sources of support.

Arthritis Research Campaign

www.arc.org.uk/

Tel: 0870 850 5000

This UK charity produces a wide range of factsheets and information booklets on all aspects of living with arthritis. Their website offers an extensive selection of links to other sources of research and support.

National Osteoporosis Society

www.nos.org.uk/

Tel: 0845 4500 230 (medical enquiries)

This UK charity's excellent website has a good section on how to keep your bones healthy and prevent the disease developing. There's also plenty of other information and links to support groups around the UK.

Alzheimer's Society

www.alzheimers.org.uk/

Tel: 020 7306 0606

A very clear and accessible website offering a wealth of information and support for sufferers of Alzheimer's, and their friends, families or carers, along with useful tips and advice on how to tailor your lifestyle to prevent the disease.

Index

Page numbers in *italic* refer to illustrations

acne 92–6, 92, 99
addiction: to drugs 56
          to exercise 60–1
adrenal glands *61*, 62, 73, 79
adrenaline *61*, 62, 73, 79–80, 114, 132
ageing 85, 96–100, 97, 146–9
AIDS 131
air travel 80–1
alcohol 21–31, 51, 52, 56, 63
          cancer prevention 138, 142–3
          cutting down 30–1, 152
          detoxing 45, 48
          fertility problems 122
          hangovers 26–7
          and heart disease 135
          intoxication 23–6
allergies 21
Alzheimer's disease 148–9
amygdala 114, *114*
angina 132
anorexia nervosa 44, 123
antibiotics 19, 88, 95
anxiety 65–6
arterial disease 132
arthritis 127, 146, 147
aspirin 81, 88
Atkins diet 35, 40–1

baldness 102–5, *102*
beards 104
biological clocks 72–3, 83, 122
blood clots 81–3, 132
blood pressure 132, 135
blood sugar levels 41, 158
body fat 34–5, 44–5, *44*
body image 105–9
body-mass index (BMI) 34, 123

body odour 100–1
bones, osteoporosis 127, 147, 148
bowel cancer 139–40
brain: Alzheimer's disease 148–9
          depression 67–9
          effects of drugs 52–6, *55*
          exercise and 58, *58*
          pleasure 56, 115
          and relationships 114–16, *114*, 116
          SCN (master body-clock) 72–3, *72*, 79, 83
          stress 62, 65
breast cancer 140–3, 156
breathing 63

caffeine 45, 48, 63, 78, 122
calcium 147, 148
calories 12–13, 17, 33, 34, 40
cancer 127, 136–45
          breast cancer 140–3, 156
          cervical cancer 143–4
          colon cancer 139–40, 156
          lung cancer 134, 136–9
          preventing 138, 156
          prostate cancer 145–6
          skin cancer 85, 97, 159
          testicular cancer 144–5
cannabis 52, 54, 56
carbohydrates 13–17, 40–1, 158
cervical cancer 143–4
chlamydia 119, 128–9, *129*
cholesterol *12*, 132, 135
circadian rhythms 72–3, *72*, 83
clothes, and body odour 101
cocaine 52, 53, 54, 56, 115
collagen 96, 97
colon cancer 139–40, 156
colonic irrigation 46, *47*
comfort food 43
condoms 88, 131, 144

contraception 117, 144
contraceptive pill 88, 140–2, 143–4
cortisol *61*, 62–5, 68, 73, 79–80, 124
cosmetic surgery 105–9
cosmetics, anti-ageing products 97–100
cravings 21

deep vein thrombosis (DVT) 81–3
dehydration 81–2, 87, 88, 152
deodorants 101
depression 66–9
detox diets 43–9
DHT, and hair loss *102*, 103
diaries 40
diarrhoea 87, 88
diet 11–21
          cancer protection 138
          detox diets 43–9
          fertility problems 124
          food labels 16
          and heart disease 132
          supplements 17–18, 19
          weight loss 33–43
dopamine 55–6, *55*, 68, 115
driving, tiredness and 76
drugs: anti-baldness treatments 103–5
          fertility treatments 125
          recreational drugs 51, 52–8, 115, 122
dry-brushing, lymphatic massage 48

eating disorders 61, 105, 123
ecstasy 52, 54
eggs, fertilization 119, 125
elastin 96, *97*
emotions, love 114–15
endorphins 58, *58*, 116–17
exercise 160–1
          addiction to 60–1

cancer protection 138
detoxing 48
and heart disease 132, 134–5
mood-lifting properties 58–9
protecting bones 147
and stress 63
weight loss 42

fasting 45
fats, dietary 13, 17, 134, 149, 155
    see also body fat; weight
fertility 117–25, 129
fibre 14, 139–40
'fight or flight' response 61, 62, 65,
    79–80
finasteride 103, 104–5
fish 134, 149
folic acid 124, 140, 149
food see diet
food intolerance 21
food poisoning 87
free radicals 85
fruit 14, 48, 134, 140, 146, 147,
    149, 156

genes 112–13, 136, 142, 144
genital herpes 128, 130–1, 130
genital warts 128, 131, 143
gonorrhoea 128, 129

hair loss 102–5, 102
hangovers 26–7
health care 127–49, 162–3
heart disease 44, 45, 64, 127,
    132–5, 142, 149, 156
heroin 52, 54–5, 56
herpes simplex virus (HSV) 128,
    130–1, 130
high blood pressure 132, 135
HIV 128, 131
holidays 80–8
homocysteine 134, 149
hormone replacement therapy (HRT)
    142–3
hormones: and acne 92, 96
    and attraction 114–15, 114
    and body fat 44–5, 44
    circadian rhythms 72–3, 72
    effects of alcohol 24–5
    and hair loss 102, 103
    menopause 135
    stress 61, 62, 79–80, 124
human papilloma virus (HPV) 128,
    131, 143
hunger 18–21, 41

illness, avoiding 127–49, 162–3
immune system 45, 48, 61, 65, 80,
    85, 112–13
infertility 119–25, 129
insomnia 80
insulin 13–17, 79, 158

jet lag 82, 83
joints, arthritis 146, 147

Kegel exercises 164

labels, food 16
lice, pubic 128
love 111–16
lung cancer 134, 136–9
lymph system 43, 45–6, 48, 49

melanin 83–5, 84, 84
melatonin 72–3, 72, 78, 79, 80, 82
men: body fat 44–5
    depression 67
    effects of alcohol 24–5
    hair loss 102–5, 102
menopause 45, 135, 148
metabolism 17, 18, 76–9, 80
minerals 17–18, 19, 149
minoxidil 103, 104–5
moisturizers 99–100
moles 85, 162

nicotine 56, 78, 122, 132, 136–9
noradrenaline 114
nutrition see diet

obesity 33, 34, 123
oestrogen 45, 115, 124, 135, 140,
    142, 148
olive oil 14, 155
omega-3 oils 134, 149
organic food 43, 48
osteoarthritis 147
osteoporosis 127, 147, 148
overweight see weight
ovulation 25, 119, 123, 124, 140
oxytocin 115

panic attacks 66
parasites 128
pelvic inflammatory disease 119,
    129, 129
pelvic-floor exercises 164
pineal gland 72–3, 72, 79
pituitary gland 58, 58, 62, 73
portion sizes 41

pregnancy 44, 45, 117–25, 129
prostate cancer 145–6
protein 13, 14, 17
pubic lice 128

relationships 111–17, 124
relaxation 63, 71, 80
restaurants 14
retinoic acid 99

salt 14, 134
saturated fats 134, 149, 155
scabies 128
sebaceous glands 92, 95
self-esteem 42, 59, 61
serotonin 67–8
sex 111, 114–15, 117, 123–4, 164
sexually transmitted infections (STIs)
    128–31, 129
shoes 101
skin: acne 92–6, 92, 99
    cancer 85, 97, 159
    sun protection 83–7, 84, 96–7,
        98, 100, 138, 159
    wrinkles 96–100, 97
sleep 48, 63, 71, 73–80
smear tests 143, 144, 163
smoking 63, 78
    and cancer 136–9, 143, 144
    detoxing 45, 48
    fertility problems 122
    and heart disease 132, 134
    and osteoporosis 147
    quitting 154
    skin damage 96
    and weight control 105
sperm 25, 119, 122–3, 125
stress 61–5, 79–80, 124
strokes 64, 65, 127, 132, 156
sugars 13–17, 41, 158
suicide 68–9
sun damage, skin 83–7, 84, 96–7,
    98, 98, 100, 138, 159
sunburn 85, 159
supplements 17–18, 19
surgery, cosmetic 105–9
sweat glands 100–1
syphilis 128, 130

testicles 121, 122–3, 129
testicular cancer 144–5
testosterone 44, 115, 124
thirst 41
tiredness 76
tomatoes 146

toxins, detox diets 43–9
travel 80–8
treats 41–2, 49

ultraviolet rays 84–5, *84*, 86–7, 96–7,
   98, 100, 159

vegetables 14, 48, 134, 140, 146,
   147, 149, 156
vitamins 17–18, 19, 149

waist measurement 34
warts, genital 128, 131, 143
water, drinking 41, 48, 81, 87, 152
weight: body image 105
   body-mass index (BMI) 34, 123
   diets 33–43
   health risks 34
   and infertility 123
   weighing yourself 42
women: body fat 44–5, *44*
   depression 67
   effects of alcohol 24–5
   heart disease 135
worry 65–6
wrinkles 85, 96–100, *97*

yo-yo dieting 38

Acknowledgements

We would like to thank all those at BBC Worldwide who helped bring this book to life, particularly Emma Shackleton, our Commissioning Editor, for her clear vision and support throughout, and Sarah Miles, whose hard work and constant enthusiasm for the project has meant so much to us. Thanks too to Annette Peppis for her thoughtful work on the design and layout and to Alan Burton for the illustrations.

The idea to write this book grew out of the BBC3 series *Body Hits*. Stuart Murphy (Controller, BBC3), Seetha Kumar and Sarah Hargreaves were all instrumental in getting it on the air. A very big thank you also to Judith Bunting (Executive Producer, *Body Hits*) for her encouragement as we drafted the text. Thanks are also due to Phil Dolling, producers Andy Robbins, Helen Seaman, Steve Crabtree, Nicola Cook, Paul King, VJ Anderson, Tracy Mason, Paul Olding and all the researchers on the team whose hard work on the series also helped us to get the words down on paper.

John would like to thank Marnie Jung and Joanna Kaye at KBJ Management for their advice and enthusiasm throughout and a big thank you from both of us to our family and friends for all their support. Cheers to you all!

Picture Credits

BBC Worldwide would like to thank the following for permission to reproduce copyright material. While every effort has been made to trace and acknowledge all copyright holders, we would like to apologize for any errors or omissions.

Alamy 57, 141; BBC Good Food Magazine 135; Corbis 70, 74–5, 89; Getty Images 6, 9, 10, 15, 20, 29, 31, 32, 39, 50, 64, 90, 109, 110, 113, 126, 150, 160–1, 163; Photonica 153, 157; Retna 117 (Philip Reeson); Vichy 98; Zefa 149.

Illustrations by Alan Burton.